Mehrshad Jafari

The Role of Biochemistry of Hormones & Heredity in Hereditary Diseases

Mehrshad Jafari

The Role of Biochemistry of Hormones & Heredity in Hereditary Diseases

Based on the Points of Pharmacology & Biochemistry

Noor Publishing

Imprint

Any brand names and product names mentioned in this book are subject to trademark, brand or patent protection and are trademarks or registered trademarks of their respective holders. The use of brand names, product names, common names, trade names, product descriptions etc. even without a particular marking in this work is in no way to be construed to mean that such names may be regarded as unrestricted in respect of trademark and brand protection legislation and could thus be used by anyone.

Cover image: www.ingimage.com

Publisher:
Noor Publishing
is a trademark of
Dodo Books Indian Ocean Ltd. and OmniScriptum S.R.L publishing group

120 High Road, East Finchley, London, N2 9ED, United Kingdom
Str. Armeneasca 28/1, office 1, Chisinau MD-2012, Republic of Moldova, Europe
Printed at: see last page
ISBN: 978-620-5-63428-8

The Role of Biochemistry of Hormones & Heredity in Hereditary Diseases Based on the Points of Pharmacology & Biochemistry

By

Mehrshad Jafari

PhD of Biochemistry-Molecular Cell

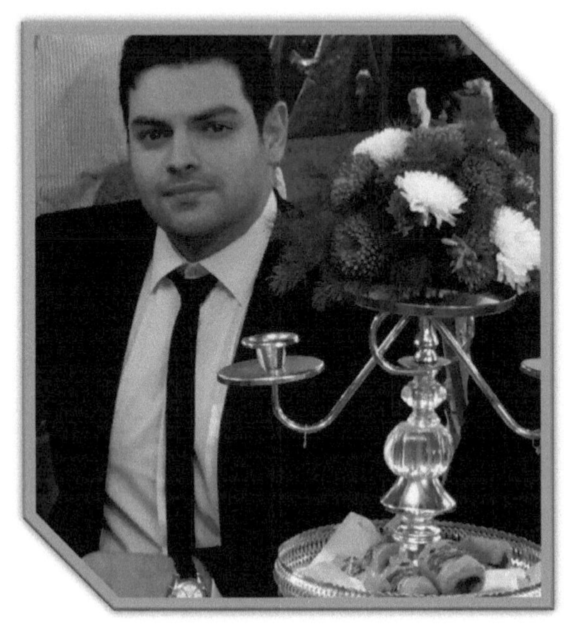

Mehrshad Jafari

PhD of Biochemistry-Molecular Cell

Dedicated to the merciful angels who:

The lord of the worlds, who began to guide his servants with the teaching of the pen.

My parents, whose presence is a crown of honor for me and their name is a reason for my existence because these two existences after the lord, have been the source of my existence, took my hand and taught me to walk in this valley full of ups and downs.

Content

Chapter I

Introduction

Introduction

What is a hormone?

Endocrine glands, which are different in the body of living organisms, release their secretions, which are called hormones, into the blood. These chemicals are transported to the target organs (groups of cells that are specific to the effect of a particular hormone) and convey their message to these cells. Controlling the cells of the body through hormones is simple in single-celled organisms, but in the body of complex organisms such as humans, it requires a complex function. Examples of these messages are blood sugar regulation, bone growth, etc. The word hormone, which is Greek, means "I arouse".

What is a hormone?

How body hormones work

To respond to specific stimulation in the body, hormones are secreted and the desired message is sent to the target cell and its connection is done through receptors on the target cell. The receptors of the target cells are proteins and can be membrane or intracellular. In other words, the connection is made in the same membrane or it goes inside the cell. These receptors are three dimensional and act like locks and keys by binding to hormones. After connecting, it executes the command it had in that cell and by performing new reactions, it causes changes in the cells. Hormones either control a specific part of the body or are in charge of general control.

Transfer of hormones in the body

According to their type, hormones are transported in the blood free or bound with specific proteins. For example, peptide hormones are transported in a soluble form in plasma, and steroid and thyroid hormones are transferred in connection with plasma proteins. Hormones are inactive when they are attached to these proteins. These hormones are transferred in the blood at a slower rate and remain in the blood for a long time (several hours or days). This time is 20 to 100 days for steroid hormones and one to six days for thyroid hormones.

Transfer of hormones in the body

Types of hormones

Based on their structure, body hormones are divided into four categories: peptide, amino, steroid and prostanoid. Peptide hormones can be simple peptides (like insulin), or they can be glycopeptides (like LH, FSH).

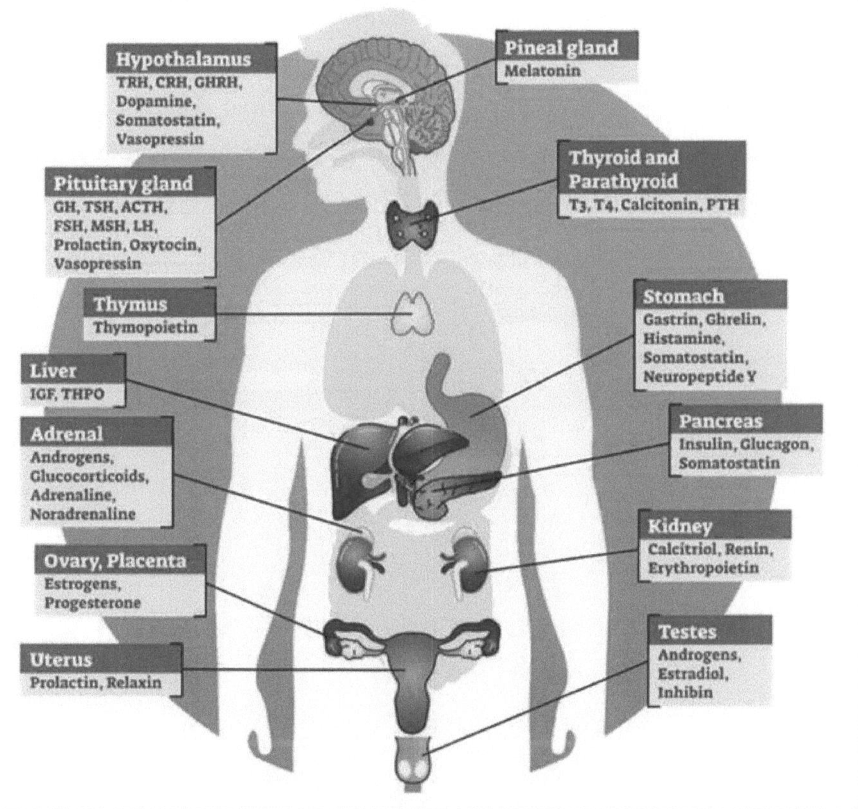

Figure 1. What are Hormones?

Steroid hormones such as sex hormones (estrogen, testosterone) have cholesterol origin. Amino hormones (such as thyroid hormones) are made up of one amino acid. Prostanoid hormones, which are not classified as hormones in some categories, are derived from unsaturated fatty acids. Hormones can also be classified based on the organs that produce them. Hypothesis, thyroid, adrenal gland hormones, etc. are examples of them. Steroid and thyroid hormones can cross the membrane and enter the cell, but peptide hormones cannot cross the membrane.

Types of hormones

Cells secreting hormones

Endocrine system is a system from which hormones are secreted and it can be a gland, an organ or a cell of an organ. Endocrine glands include pituitary gland, hypothalamus, ovary, testicles, thyroid, parathyroid, adrenal gland, thymus, and pineal gland. Organs that secrete hormones are pancreas, liver and kidneys. The pituitary gland is a gland that regulates the amount of hormone secretion by other glands and how they work.

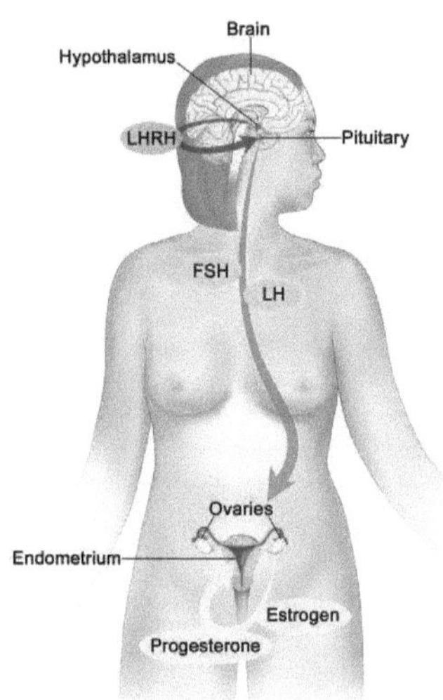

Figure 2. Female Hormone Loop: Image Details

The hormones secreted by the hypothalamus gland control the release of hormones such as sleep and control body temperature and hunger. The secretion of sex hormones and cortisol is from the adrenal gland. Insulin is one of the important hormones in the body that lowers blood sugar and is produced by the pancreas. The testes produce and secrete male hormones (sperm and testosterone) and the ovaries produce and secrete female hormones (testosterone and progesterone). Hormones secreted by the thyroid gland control the amount of calories the body uses. The parathyroid gland also controls blood and bone calcium.

Regulating the release of hormones in the body

The amount of hormone secretion, which is controlled by the nervous system, is influenced by the concentration of hormones in the blood. Regulating the amount of hormone secretion with the amount of hormones itself is called self-regulation, which exists in two forms, positive and negative. In one type, when the amount of hormone in the blood is high, its secretion decreases.

For example, by eating food and eliminating hunger, the secretion of ghrelin hormone that was secreted during hunger decreases, and it is called negative self-regulation. But in its own positive regulation, the high amount and concentration of hormones in the blood, such as the hormone oxytocin (love hormone), increases its secretion and production.

The work of some body hormones

In this section, the function of some hormones in the body is introduced, for example, the hormone estrogen is responsible for regulating the period in women and controlling sexual stimulation in women and men. Progesterone is the hormone that changes the body and prepares it for pregnancy, and estriol is the sex hormone that grows the uterus and prepares it for childbirth. Insulin lowers blood sugar. Serotonin is responsible for controlling sleep and appetite. During intense emotions, the hormone adrenaline is released and gives a person more energy. LH is a hormone that controls the reproductive system in men and women.

Hormonal diseases

Hormones are secreted and produced from the endocrine glands and continue their regulatory process with natural secretion. But when, for any reason, the secretion of these hormones and the work of these glands are disrupted, the hormonal balance is disturbed and causes various diseases. Some of these diseases are described below.

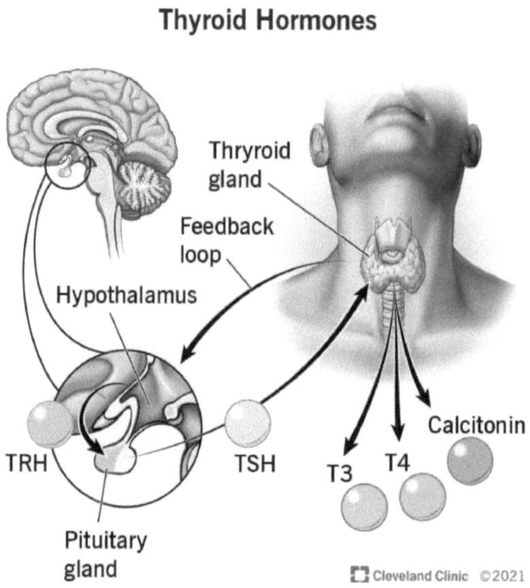

Thyroid Hormones

Thryroid gland

Feedback loop

Hypothalamus

TRH TSH T3 T4 Calcitonin

Pituitary gland

Cleveland Clinic ©2021

Figure 3. Thyroid Hormone: What It Is & Function

Diabetes

This type of disease occurs when the body uses the insulin hormone incorrectly and disrupts the balance of this hormone, which can even affect the function of other hormones such as thyroid and cortisol.

Hypothyroidism or hyperthyroidism

Thyroxine hormone, which is released from the thyroid gland, causes hypothyroidism if it is produced in a small amount, and hyperthyroidism if it is produced in a large amount. Hypothyroidism causes fatigue, depression and decreased heart rate, and hyperthyroidism causes weight loss and insomnia. In general, this hormone regulates the correct use of calories by the body and is responsible for the activity of various organs such as the heart and brain.

Addison's disease

Cortisol is not produced enough in the body of people with Addison's disease, and even aldosterone may not be produced enough and the body of these patients undergoes changes. Low blood pressure, fatigue and low blood sugar are symptoms of this disease.

Turner syndrome

In this genetic disease, which is specific to women, one of the X chromosomes is lost. These people have late puberty and slow growth.

Congenital adrenal hyperplasia

In these patients, one of the enzymes of the adrenal gland is lost. Hormones secreted from this gland control the immune system, blood pressure and body metabolism.

The amount of hormones in the body

The amount of hormones in the blood is very low, about one Pico gram (one millionth of a millionth of a gram) to several micrograms (a millionth of a gram) in one milliliter of blood. What role do hormones play in the body and what effects do they have on our body? Estrogen, progesterone, testosterone, prolactin and FSH / LH are among the important hormones in the body that have a great impact on our menstruation, fertility, sexual desire, mental state, sleep cycle and appetite. The reactivation of reproductive system hormones can affect menstruation, fertility and sexual desire, and even your mental state, sleep cycle, and appetite. Here we discuss some hormones that cause such disorders.

If it hits you once a month and you run out of the house at 2 O'clock in the morning and look for a sweet shop, guess what happened to you? You are a natural. The reactivation of hormones in the reproductive system can affect menstruation, fertility and libido, and even your mental state, sleep cycle and appetite. Here we discuss some hormones that cause such disorders.

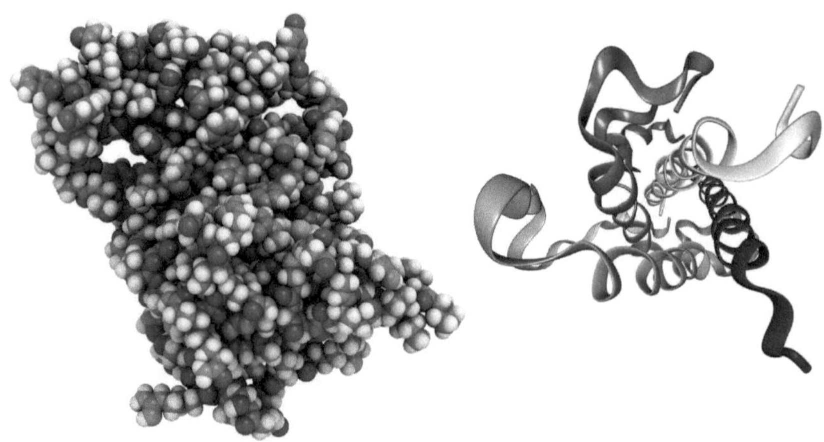

Figure 4. Definition, Function, & Types

Estrogen

Estradiol (or female sex hormone) actually prepares the uterus for fertilization. Its balanced and constant amount can increase the strength and libido and the functioning of the immune system.

Main effects: Estrogen sends "Growth" signals to every cell in the body, from breasts to bones. But its high amount can lead to premenstrual syndrome and even breast cancer, which is the enemy of fertility. Its low amount can also lead to osteoporosis.

Balancing activity: Being too thin can interfere with the production of this hormone, on the other hand, too many fat cells produce a type of estrogen that, along with estradiol, causes problems in the body's internal system. The solution is to have a balanced and proportionate weight. Try to have your body mass index between 18.5 and 30.

Progesterone

Progesterone builds the inner lining of the uterus (that is, the bed or place of the embryo) every month.

Main effects: Progesterone has a mild sedative effect that can lead to a good and comfortable sleep. On the other hand, it can increase water retention, bloating and constipation.

Balancing activity: Since the regulation of this hormone is very important for the formation of the fetus, many mothers who wish to have children turn to the use of over-the-counter creams. It is recommended not to do this. Research has shown that these creams have no benefit. What can work for you is five minutes of meditation a day.

Testosterone

This androgen hormone can cover your regular ovulation and your hot sex drive.

Main effects: Very high levels – often associated with polycystic ovary syndrome – can lead to acne, dandruff or the growth of dark hair in unusual areas of the body. On the other hand, its deficiency can reduce your strength and sexual desire and your health.

Balancing activity: High testosterone is closely related to obesity. So try to keep your body mass index in balance. If this index is low, eating zinc-rich foods such as hummus can increase its amount.

Prolactin

This hormone is produced in the brain and its main job is to control the release of eggs and stimulate milk production in mothers who have just given birth.

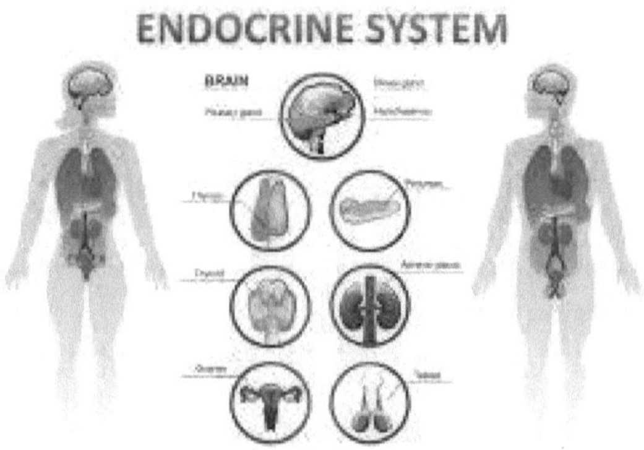

Figure 5. Patient Engagement, Endocrine Society

Main effects: It's very high amount in rare cases can disrupt your libido and lead to symptoms similar to menopause symptoms. A slight increase in the amount of this hormone affects ovulation. After giving birth, the balanced amount of this hormone will help you lose weight faster.

Balancing activity: Sleep disturbance increases the level of stress hormones, such as cortisol and prolactin. With seven to eight hours of continuous and balanced sleep, this hormone will be at its balanced level.

FSH / LH

Lymph gland stimulating hormone (FHS) prepares the eggs for the first time and luteinizing hormone (LH) decreases it.

Main effects: The optimal amount of FSH / LH can also cause a balanced amount of progesterone in conditions where its increase is associated with memory problems, insomnia and acne.

What is hormonal imbalance?

When a hormonal imbalance occurs, it means that the amount of a certain hormone in the body is too much or too little. Even small changes can have serious effects on your entire body. Look at hormones like a cake recipe. As you know, the increase or decrease of each element in the preparation of raw materials and cooking affects the final product. Of course, sometimes due to aging, there are interferences and fluctuations in the body's hormones, which are considered normal due to aging.

Symptoms of hormonal imbalance

Your hormones play an essential role in your overall health. For this reason, there is a wide range of symptoms that can be a sign of hormonal imbalance. Your symptoms depend on which hormones or glands are malfunctioning.

Common hormonal conditions that affect both men and women can cause any of the following symptoms

➤ Weight Gain;

➤ Fatigue;

➤ Increased sensitivity to cold or heat;

➤ Constipation or frequent bowel movements;

➤ Unexplained weight loss (sometimes sudden);

➤ Increased or decreased heart rate;

➤ Muscle pain, tenderness and stiffness;

➤ Thin hair or fine and fragile hair;

➤ Increased hunger;

➤ Depression, anxiety or irritability;

➤ Blurred vision;

➤ Sweating;

➤ Sterility.

Symptoms in women

In women, the most common hormonal imbalance is polycystic ovary syndrome (PCOS). Your normal hormonal cycle also changes naturally during

- Puberty;
- Pregnancy;
- Breast feeding;
- Menopause.

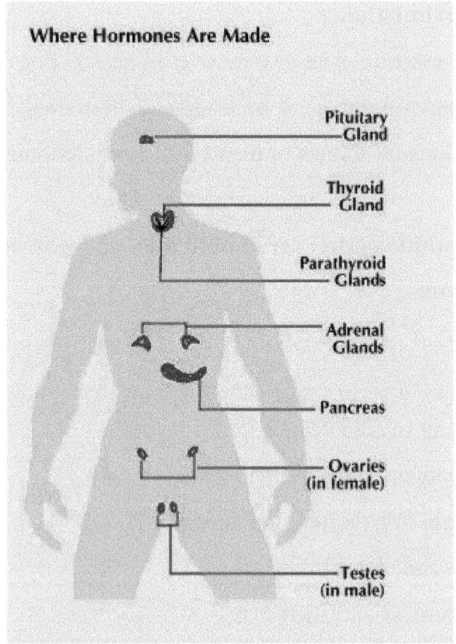

Figure 6. Hormones and their functions, Britannica

Some of the symptoms of hormonal imbalance specific to women include the following

- Irregular menstrual periods, such as a stopped period or frequent periods;
- Excess hair on the face, chin or other parts of the body;
- Acne on the face, chest or back;
- Thinning of hair or hair loss;

- ➢ Weight gain or weight loss;
- ➢ Darkening of the skin, especially along the neck, in the groin and under the breasts;
- ➢ Vaginal dryness and atrophy.

Symptoms in men

Testosterone plays an important role in male development. Not producing enough testosterone can cause various symptoms.

In adult men, symptoms include

- ➢ Breast growth;
- ➢ Erectile dysfunction;
- ➢ Loss of muscle mass;
- ➢ Sterility; and Beard reduction and body hair growth;
- ➢ Osteoporosis, loss of bone mass;
- ➢ Difficulty concentrating;
- ➢ Hot flashes.

Causes of hormonal imbalance

There are many possible causes of hormonal imbalance. Causes vary depending on what hormones or glands are affected. The main causes of hormonal imbalance are

- ➢ Diabetes;
- ➢ Hypothyroidism or hyperthyroidism;
- ➢ Hypogonadism: Gonads include testicles in men and ovaries in women. Hypogonadism is when the gonads produce less or no sex hormones.
- ➢ Cushing's syndrome: A syndrome that occurs due to high levels of the hormone cortisol.
- ➢ Tumors (benign or cancerous);
- ➢ Congenital adrenal hyperplasia;
- ➢ Medicines.

Testing and diagnosis

There is no single test available to diagnose hormonal imbalance. Depending on the symptoms, the doctor may suggest one or more diagnostic tests.

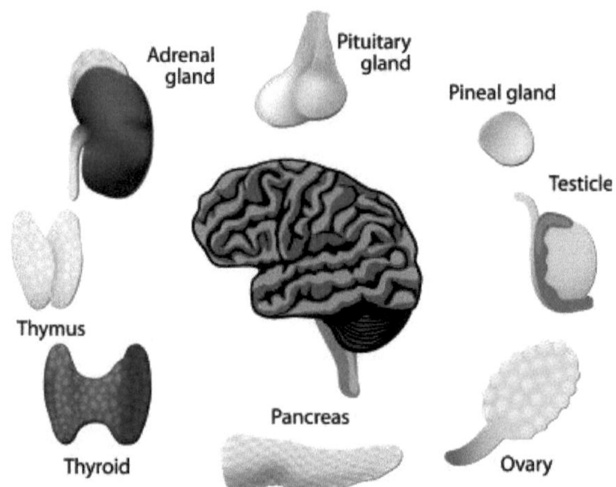

Figure 7. All About Hormones: How they Function to Keep You Healthy - Ask The Scientists

Blood test

A blood test is one of the most common methods of testing hormone levels. This test can detect testosterone, estrogen, cortisol and thyroid levels.

Pelvic test

In women, the doctor may use a pap smear scan to detect unusual masses, cysts, or tumors. In men, the doctor may check for any lumps or abnormalities.

Sonography

Doctors may use ultrasound to take pictures of the uterus, ovaries, testicles, thyroid gland, or pituitary gland. Sometimes more advanced tests are needed, such as biopsy, MRI, thyroid scan, sperm count.

Interpretation of hormonal factors in blood tests

In this section, we examine and interpret hormonal factors including estrogen, progesterone, testosterone, cortisol and prolactin.

Estrogen hormone

Estrogen is the name of a group of female sex hormones. The estrogen test measures all three types of this hormone: estrone (E1), estradiol (E2) and estriol (E3).

Low estrogen levels may be a sign of polycystic ovary syndrome (PCOS), decreased pituitary function (hypopituitarism), low testosterone (hypogonadism), anorexia nervosa, or low body fat. High estrogen levels may be associated with conditions such as obesity, diabetes, and high blood pressure.

Progesterone hormone

Progesterone is produced by the ovaries during ovulation. Its function is to help prepare the uterus to receive a fertilized egg. Persistently high progesterone levels may indicate an increased risk of breast cancer. Ovarian insufficiency is one of the causes of low progesterone levels. Also, low progesterone levels during pregnancy often predict miscarriage and premature birth. By evaluating the progesterone level, the cause of infertility or the risk of miscarriage can be predicted.

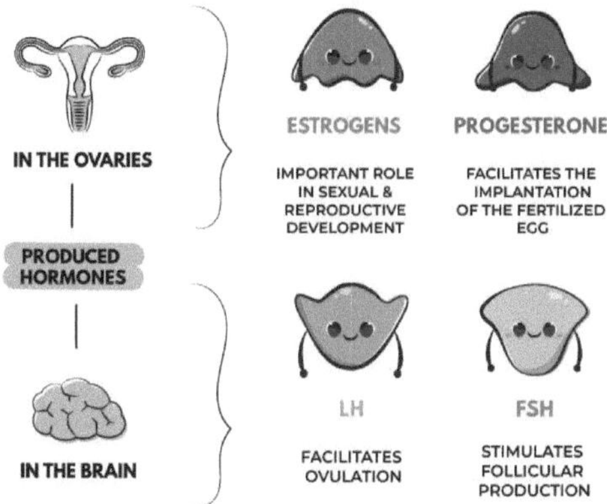

Figure 8. Female Hormones: How do they function?

Testosterone hormone

Although testosterone is commonly known as the "Male sex hormone," women also produce it. High testosterone levels may lead to irregular periods, weight gain, acne and infertility. In males; Hyperthyroidism, testicular tumor, adrenal cortical tumor, congenital hyperplasia of the adrenal gland can increase testosterone levels in them. In women, low testosterone may occur during menopause and lead to a serious decrease in libido.

Thyroid hormones

Thyroid function is measured and characterized by a group of hormones produced by the pituitary gland or the thyroid gland itself. Hyperthyroidism may cause weight loss, goiter and irregular menstrual periods in women. In women, hypothyroidism during pregnancy can lead to placental abruption, miscarriage, premature birth, low birth weight, and congenital thyroid problems.

FSH and LH hormones

Follicle Stimulating Hormone (FSH) and LH are measured to determine male and female infertility. FSH levels are also checked to determine the efficiency of male or female sex organs (testicles or ovaries). In males; FSH will cause the production of androgen-binding proteins as well as the maturation of sperms in the testicles. LH hormone is also used to investigate testicular dysfunction in men and to evaluate endocrine problems related to premature puberty in children.

Prolactin hormone

In women, prolactin causes lactation and in men its role is unclear. Increased prolactin levels can indicate prolactin secreting pituitary tumor, kidney failure, stress, polycystic ovary syndrome.

Chapter II

Recommendations for lifestyle changes

There are many nutritional supplements on the market that claim to treat menopause and hormonal imbalance. However, few of them can be justified by scientific evidence. Some people find that yoga helps treat symptoms of hormonal imbalance. Yoga is great for increasing strength, flexibility and balance. It may also help you lose weight, which in itself can help regulate your hormones.

Hormones are a group of chemicals that are produced in very small amounts in the body and have regulatory effects to maintain the normal state of the body. A decrease or increase in the amount of these hormones can cause some important diseases in humans. Hormones are secreted from special glands in the body. Sex hormones are mainly made from cholesterol in the sex glands (ovaries and testicles). These hormones are also produced in small amounts in other tissues such as adrenal glands, placenta, liver, etc. The imbalance of sex hormones leads to various diseases such as premature puberty, femininity syndromes, infertility and lack of secondary sexual characteristics.

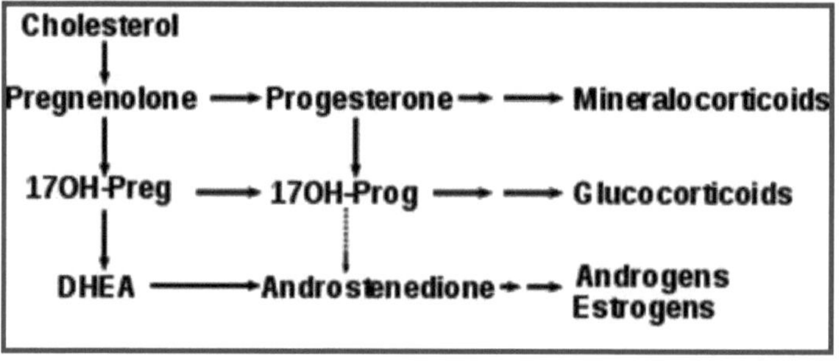

Female hormones

Estrogen

It refers to a group of hormones including estriol, estradiol and estrone that are produced in women's bodies. Estrogens are mainly produced in the ovaries, testicles and adrenals from the androgens androstenedione and testosterone. In women, estrogen is released from the egg in the follicular phase of the normal ovarian cycle. This hormone causes the growth of the female reproductive system and the development of female characteristics such as the enlargement of the breasts in the female sex and having a delicate female voice. The amount of secretion of this hormone is very low during childhood, and during puberty, their secretion increases and causes the appearance of sexual characteristics in women. Estrogens also increase the activity of bone formation and make the distribution of fat in the body more feminine (mostly in the breasts, hips and thighs).

Estrogen in the uterine wall causes the growth and hyperemia of the endometrium (inner wall of the uterus). It also reduces the release of gonad stimulating hormone in the hypothalamus and reduces the release of FSH and LH from the pituitary gland. After menopause, almost no estrogen is produced in the body, so bone building activity in the body is greatly reduced. If this condition is severe, it leads to osteoporosis in women after menopause. Estrogen measurement in cases of estrogen level evaluation in patients with abnormal menstrual cycle, abnormal excessive bleeding, checking sexual maturity, infertility, the presence of female characteristics (gynecomastia), monitoring hormone replacement therapy during menopause, as a tumor marker (diagnosis Estrogen-producing tumors) and checking ovarian function are used.

Estradiol (17-beta estradiol)

Estradiol (E2) is produced in the ovaries. Women have a retrograde mechanism for this hormone, so that the decrease in E2 levels stimulates the hypothalamus and gonadotropin-releasing factors, which stimulates the pituitary gland and releases FSH and LH hormones. These hormones stimulate the ovaries and produce E2. The amount of this hormone reaches its maximum during the ovulation phase of the monthly cycle. A small amount of this hormone is also produced in men; About one third of estrogen in the testicles and the rest of it comes from the conversion of testosterone and estrone in the surrounding tissues. A large amount of estradiol in serum is bound to albumin and sex hormone-binding globulin (SHBG), and only 2-3% exists in free form.

- Estradiol is the most abundant estrogen in premenopausal women.
- The amount of serum estradiol is different at different hours of the day and night, so in repeated tests, sampling should be done at a certain time of the day and night.
- Decreased estradiol levels are observed in ovarian failure, Turner syndrome, hypothyroidism, Stein-Lenthal syndrome, menopause, anorexia nervosa, polycystic ovary syndrome, hypothesis and hypogonadism.
- Increased estradiol levels are seen in ovarian, testicular, and adrenal tumors, early puberty in women, gynecomastia (female syndrome in men), and liver necrosis and cirrhosis.
- Contraceptive pills and clomiphene decrease serum E2 levels.
- Adrenocorticosteroids, ampicillin, drugs containing estrogen, phenothiazines and tetracycline's may increase E2 levels.

Normal values

Children under 10 years: < 15 pg./ml
Adult men: 10-50 pg./ml

Adult women

Follicular phase: 25-350 pg./ml

Mid-cycle: 150-750 pg./ml

Luteal phase: 30-450 pg./ml

After menopause: ≤ 20 pg./ml

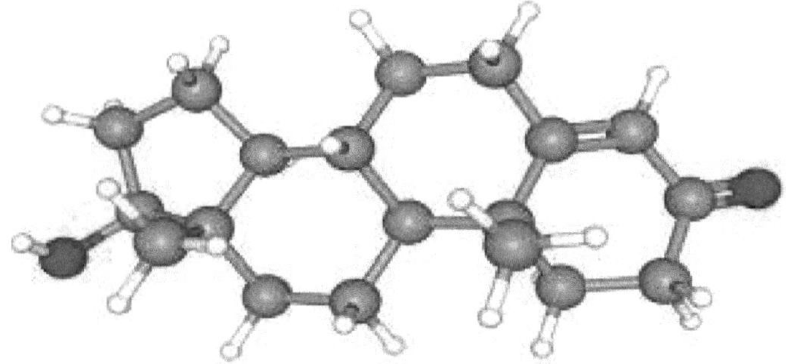

Figure 9. The Hormones

Estrone

Estrone (E1) is a weaker estrogen than estradiol that is secreted by the ovary. Also, most of estrone comes from the conversion of androstenedione in peripheral tissues and estradiol metabolism. After menopause, the ovaries degenerate and the production of estrogen is done only by the adrenal gland. In postmenopausal women, estrone forms the highest amount of estrogen.

Estriol

Estriol (E3) is the main estrogen in pregnant women and is related to the health of the placenta and fetus. Estriol is produced in the adrenal gland, fetal liver and placenta. Estriol measurement is an important indicator for the health of the fetus, so that its high level indicates the optimal function of the placenta and fetus. If the level of estriol decreases, it indicates the destruction of the placenta-fetal unit, in which case the state of pregnancy should be checked.

Repeated examinations usually start at 28 to 30 weeks of pregnancy and are then repeated weekly. If needed, the number of these tests can be increased to evaluate high-risk pregnancies. In these tests, the samples are performed daily and the sample is compared to the previous sample. The amount of serum estriol is different at different hours of the day and night, so in repeated tests, sampling should be done at a certain time of the day and night.

A decrease in the amount of estriol compared to the previous sample indicates the deterioration of the fetus.

- ➢ This hormone is measured in the laboratory as free estriol, 16-hydroxyestradiol, unconjugated estriol (UE3).
- ➢ This test is used to check the health of the placenta and the fetus and to assess the risk of premature birth, and it is one of the required tests in the screening of the second trimester of pregnancy (quad marker), which is used to screen for Down syndrome, trisomy 18 and neural tube defects. Natural tube defects are used. This test is performed in the 15th week and 5 days before the 20th week of pregnancy.
- ➢ Unconjugated estriol is also used to evaluate estrogen metabolism, epidemiological studies of breast cancer along with the measurement of estrone, estradiol and various metabolites and as an element in the diagnosis of prenatal steroid metabolism disorders in fetuses such as Smith-Lemli-Opitz syndrome. X-linked acytosis and linked gene syndrome (placental sulfatase deficiency disorders), aromatase deficiency, primary and secondary adrenal insufficiency, and various forms of congenital adrenal hyperplasia are used.
- ➢ Premature birth, pre-eclampsia, anemia, severe liver disease and fetal loss cause a decrease in estriol levels.
- ➢ Its amount increases in multiple pregnancy and oxytocin consumption.

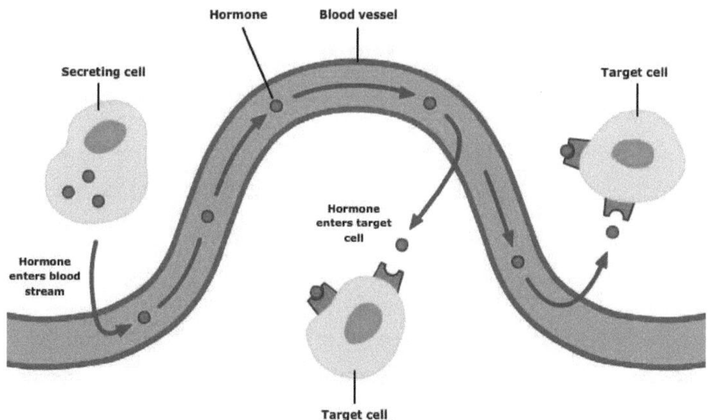

Figure 10. Hormonal control of digestion, Science Learning Hub

Normal values

Men: < 0.07 ng/ml

Women: < 0.08 ng/ml

Pregnant women

First 3 months of pregnancy: < 38 ng/ml

Second 3 months of pregnancy: 38-140 ng/ml

3rd month of pregnancy: 31-460 ng/ml

Progesterone

Progesterone is a hormone that is secreted in a small amount from the adrenal glands and more from the corpus luteum in the ovary. Progesterone causes the growth and regeneration of the inner lining of the uterus and prepares the uterus to replace the fertilized egg.

After ovulation, the level of progesterone in the plasma increases; The corpus luteum produces and secretes a large amount of progesterone. If fertilization does not take place, the corpus luteum will be destroyed; Therefore, the loss of the corpus luteum, which is the main source of progesterone production, will cause a drop in blood progesterone levels, which will lead to the onset of menstrual bleeding. If fertilization occurs and the fertilized egg is replaced in the uterus, the corpus luteum remains and continues to produce progesterone in the first few weeks of pregnancy. Then the corpus luteum is replaced by the placenta. From now until the end of pregnancy, the placenta will be responsible for the production and secretion of the major hormone progesterone.

The amount of progesterone and urinary concentrations of its metabolites (such as pregnanediol) increase in the second half of the normal ovulation period. Therefore, the amount of progesterone provides accurate information about the time of ovulation.

Clinical use of progesterone

- Making sure of ovulation during the menstrual cycle;
- Investigating the causes of infertility;
- Investigating the causes of abnormal vaginal bleeding;
- Assessment of placental health with frequent progesterone measurements in high-risk pregnancies;
- Monitoring the therapeutic effect of progesterone (progesterone is prescribed in early pregnancy in order to maintain pregnancy);
- Examining some patients with adrenal disorders;
- Diagnosis of ectopic pregnancy and abortion.

Attention

- Progesterone increases after ovulation, pregnancy, ovarian cysts, adrenal hyperplasia, hereditary adrenal hyperplasia, testicular tumors, ovarian carcinoma, mole pregnancy.
- Progesterone reduction occurs in pre-eclampsia, pregnancy poisoning, miscarriage, placental insufficiency, fetal death, ovarian neoplasm, amenorrhea, ovarian function reduction and ectopic pregnancy.
- Estrogen, progesterone and clomiphene drugs can interfere with the test.

➢ Hemolysis caused by improper location of the sample can affect the test results.

➢ Do not use food supplements containing biotin 12 hours before sampling.

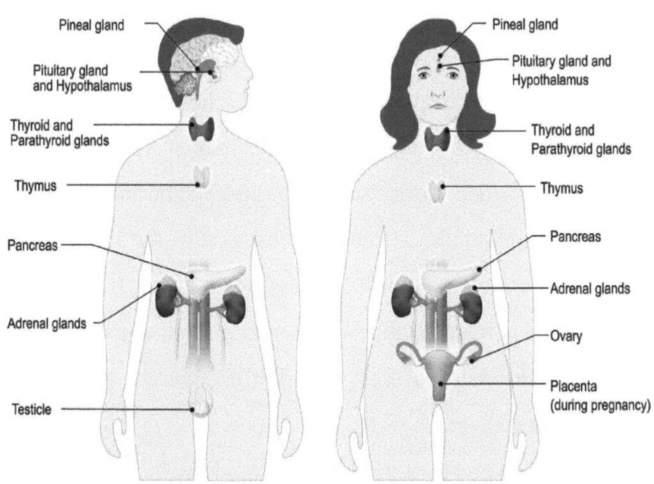

Figure 11. The Endocrine (or Hormonal) System - Hormones Australia

Normal values

Children

Less than 9 years: <20 ng/dL

10-15 years: <20 ng/dL

Men: 10-50 ng/dl

Women

Follicular phase: <50 ng/dL

Luteal phase: 300-2500 ng/dl

Menopause: <40

Pregnant women

First 3 months of pregnancy: 725-4400 ng/dL

Second 3 months of pregnancy: 1950-8250 ng/dl

3rd month of pregnancy: 6500-22900 ng/Dl

Testosterone

Testosterone is one of the important androgen hormones that stimulate spermatogenesis and secondary sexual characteristics in men. This hormone acts as a precursor to estrogen in women. Testosterone has androgenic and anabolic effects in both sexes. In men, testosterone is mostly produced in the lydic cells of the testicles and a small amount of it is made in the adrenal gland. In premenopausal women, most testosterone is made in the ovaries and a small amount of it is made in the adrenal gland and peripheral tissues. But after menopause, the amount of its production in the ovary decreases.

Testosterone production in the testes and ovaries is regulated by a pituitary negative feedback mechanism. So that an increase in serum testosterone level causes a decrease in serum LH levels, while a decrease in serum testosterone will lead to an increase in serum LH. Most of the testosterone in the blood is bound to sex hormone binding globulins (SHBG) and a small amount is bound to albumin and a small amount is free. Total testosterone levels vary throughout the day. Its highest amount is in the early morning and its lowest amount is in the afternoon.

> Total testosterone measurement is suitable for most diagnostic purposes, especially when combined with LH and FSH tests. Of course, in cases of mild testosterone homeostasis disorders such as abnormal function and SHBG level, total testosterone measurement is not enough and free testosterone should be evaluated. Free testosterone can be measured in cases of obesity, cirrhosis and thyroid disorders.

> The amount of testosterone before puberty is low in boys and it increases during puberty. This causes thickening of the voice, enlargement of muscles, production of sperm and growth of facial and body hair.

- Excessive production of this hormone in boys causes premature puberty. This condition can be caused by testicular, adrenal or pituitary tumors.
- Excessive production of this hormone in women is seen in ovarian, adrenal and adrenal gland hyperplasia, trophoblastic tumor, polycystic ovary, which causes masculinity and appears in the form of amenorrhea and hirsutism.
- The most common causes of testosterone increase are genetic factors, such as genetic hyperplasia of the adrenal gland, tumors of the adrenal, testicle and ovary, and athletes' abuse of testosterone and gonadotropins.
- Hyperthyroidism, testosterone resistance syndrome, encephalitis and hypothalamic tumor also lead to an increase in testosterone.
- Decreased testosterone in men may indicate hypogonadism, which leads to changes in secondary sexual characteristics and reproductive performance.
- Low levels of testosterone are seen in Klinefelter syndrome, liver cirrhosis, trisomy 21, hypogonadism and primary and secondary hypogonadism.
- Clomiphene, anticonvulsants, barbiturates, estrogens, and oral contraceptives increase testosterone levels.
- Androgens, dexamethasone, diethyl acetyl bestrol, digoxin, alcohol, steroids, ketoconazole, phenothiazine and spironolactone decrease testosterone levels.

Clinical application of testosterone

- Assessment of delayed puberty or early puberty in boys;
- Testosterone monitoring in alternative treatment methods;
- Testosterone monitoring in treatment with antiandrogens in diseases such as prostate cancer, premature puberty, hirsutism and male and female gender disorders.
- Investigating the cause of secondary male characteristics in women such as hair loss and amenorrhea.
- Investigation of polycystic ovary syndrome (PCOS); Patients with this an ovulatory syndrome have hirsutism, acne and male pattern hair loss.
- Diagnosis of androgen-producing tumors.

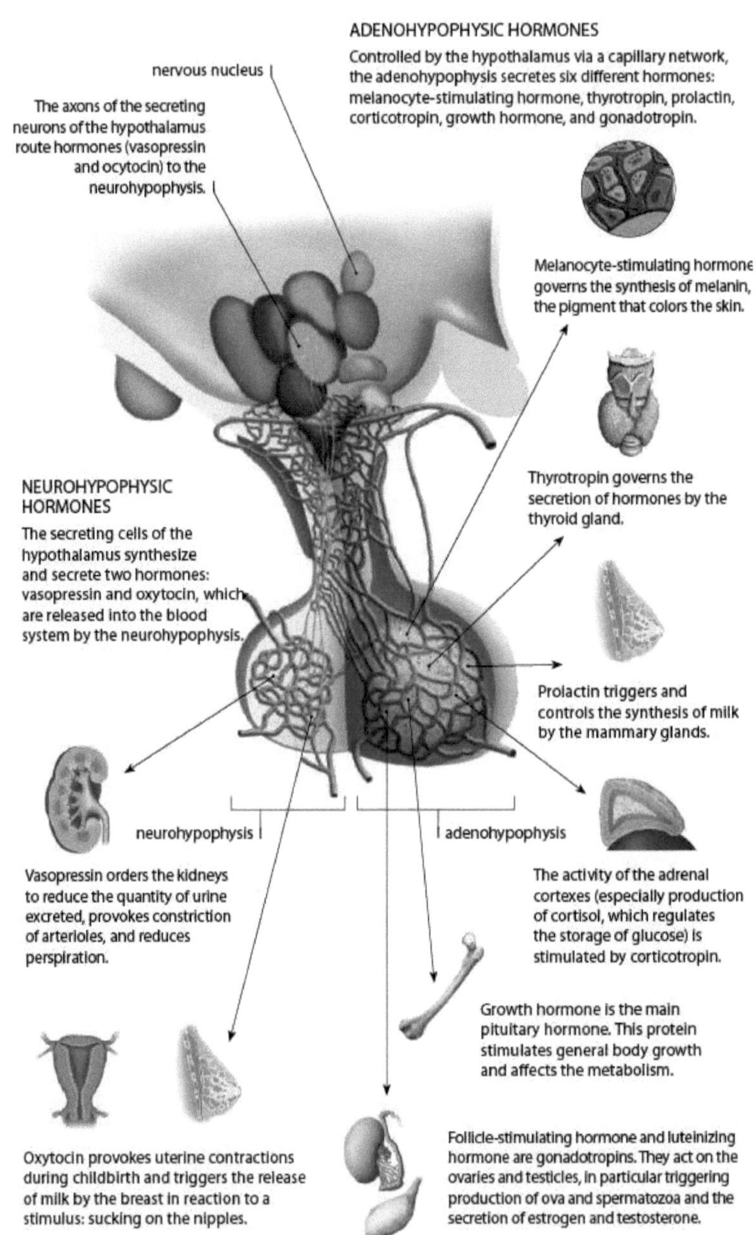

Figure 12. Hormones: the body's chemical messengers | Visual Dictionary

Normal values

Men

0-5 months: 75-400 nano grams per deciliter

6 months-9 years: > 7-20 nano grams per deciliter

10-11 years: >7-130 nano grams per deciliter

12-13 years: > 7-800 nano grams per deciliter

14 years: 7-1200 nano grams per deciliter

15-16 years: 100-1200 nano grams per deciliter

17-18 years: 300-1200 nano grams per deciliter

Equal to or more than 19 years: 240-950 nano grams per deciliter.

Women

0-5 months: 20-80 nano grams per deciliter

6 months-9 years: > 7-20 nano grams per deciliter

10-11 years: >7-44 nano grams per deciliter

12-16 years: >44-75 nano grams per deciliter

17-18 years: 20-75 nano grams per deciliter

Equal to or more than 19 years: 8-60 nano grams per deciliter

Free testosterone: 0.3-2 pg./ml

Percentage of free testosterone: 0.1-0.3%

The role of hormones in brain injury recovery

Recent studies have shown that giving certain hormones to rats without brain damage can cause motor responses similar to human motor deficits on one side of the body. According to Science Daily; A stroke or damage to one side of the brain causes movement problems on the opposite side of the body. Scientists previously thought that these movement problems were caused by nerves on one side controlling brain activity on the opposite side. But recent studies have shown that giving certain hormones to rats without brain damage can cause motor responses similar to human motor deficits on one side of the body.

Georgi Bakalkin, professor at Uppsala University's Department of Pharmaceutical Biosciences and senior author, explains that the study sought to answer one question, whether pituitary hormones can partially account for movement problems related to the side of the body experienced after brain injury. To further investigate, Bakalkin and his team investigated the effects of unilateral brain damage in rats that lacked connections between the brain and the nerves that control the hind limbs. They found that even without this connection, the contralateral limb of the injury had impaired reflexes. Animals lacking a pituitary gland did not experience these problems. It seems that two pituitary hormones - endorphin and Arg - vasopressin are involved in this disorder.

When the team gave these two hormones to mice without brain damage, the mice experienced hindlimb contractions on the right side. Next, they tested what would happen if the mice were given left brain damage drugs that blocked the effects of these two hormones. They found that the animals did not have right-sided movement problems. This suggests that after brain damage, hormones transmit specific signals, and for the treatment of patients with similar damage, the use of drugs that block these hormones can be useful. Bakalkin concludes by stating that these observations show that the endocrine system through hormones in the blood may selectively target the left and right side of the animal's body. This is an unusual phenomenon that requires further studies and confirmation in other animal models. If our future human studies confirm the benefits of this type of treatment, it will provide a new approach to treating movement problems after stroke or injury.

The role of hormones in weight control

Hormones play a major role in controlling your weight, affect your appetite, and control your body fat storage. In this article, we examine 9 hormones that play a role in weight control.

Insulin hormone

Insulin is produced by beta cells in the pancreas. The amount of this hormone increases after meals. Insulin hormone is the main fat storage hormone in the body. In patients with insulin resistance, both blood sugar and insulin levels increase dramatically, which can lead to problems such as obesity and metabolic syndrome.

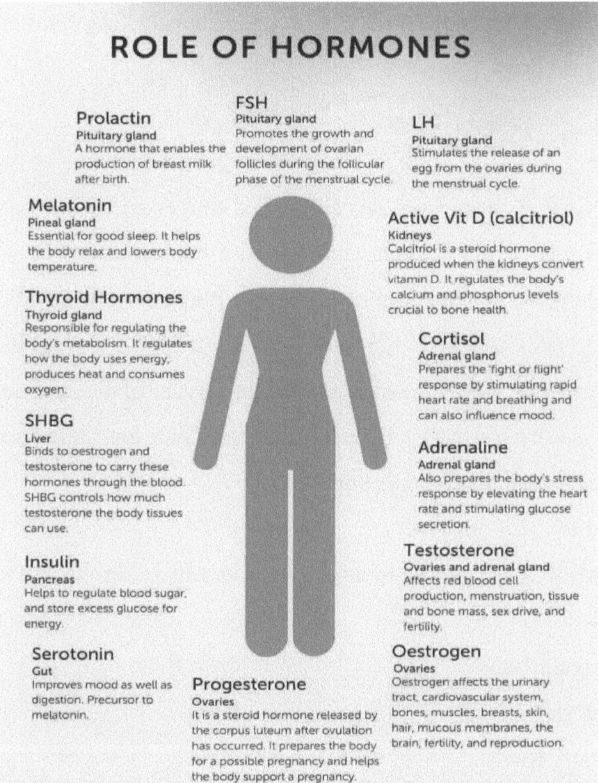

Figure 13. How Female Hormones Impact Women"s Health - Not Just Fertility

To control blood insulin levels, pay attention to the following points

➢ Reducing the consumption of sugar: Fructose and sucrose in food increases insulin secretion and insulin resistance.

➢ Reduce the consumption of carbohydrates such as white bread and white rice.

➢ Protein is one of the substances that cause insulin to rise in the short term, but in the long term, it reduces insulin resistance and is effective in shrinking the belly.

➢ Consumption of omega 3. Consumption of good fats such as omega 3 in fish.

➢ Exercise regularly.

➢ Be sure to include magnesium and related supplements in your diet.

➢ Don't forget to drink green tea.

Leptin hormone

The hormone leptin is secreted from fat cells, and is connected to the hypothalamus part of the brain, which also causes your appetite to decrease. The amount of secretion of this hormone is higher in obese people (almost 4 times that of normal people), but due to resistance to leptin, it cannot have a proper control in reducing the appetite of these people. As you lose weight, levels of the hormone leptin decrease, which is why it's harder for people to stay lean long-term because the brain assumes you're hungry and tells you to eat.

Hence, it is better to:

➢ Avoid foods that cause inflammation, such as sugary drinks and trans fatty acids.

➢ Exercise regularly;

➢ Get enough sleep;

➢ Eat more fatty foods.

Ghrelin hormone

The hormone ghrelin is also called the hunger hormone. When your stomach is empty, the amount of secretion of this hormone increases. In other words, the highest amount of this hormone is before eating, and the lowest amount is after eating and when full. The level of this hormone in obese people is lower than normal and thin people. Even research shows that the amount of ghrelin hormone decreases in obese people after eating.

To control the level of this hormone, you must:

- ➤ The consumption of sugar, fructose and sugary drinks should be controlled.
- ➤ Include protein consumption especially in breakfast.

Cortisol hormone

Cortisol is secreted from the adrenal glands. Since this hormone increases during times of stress and anxiety, it is also called stress hormone and it causes obesity. The reason why people tend to eat more food during stress is the increase in the secretion of this hormone. Also, blood cortisol levels increase in people who follow strict diets.

As a result, to have a balanced amount of cortisol hormone

- ➤ Listen to soft music, get enough sleep and meditate.
- ➤ Eat a balanced diet and avoid cutting calories.

Estrogen hormone

Estrogen is the most important female sex hormone produced by the ovaries. The increase and decrease in the secretion of this hormone depending on the age, the level of health of women and the performance of other hormones, is one of the causes of obesity in women. Due to some environmental effects, obese women have more estrogen than thin women. During menopause and with the decrease in estrogen secretion, fats are stored more in the abdominal area (visceral fat), this condition can lead to insulin resistance or other diseases.

Having a balanced diet and healthy lifestyle helps to control the level of estrogen secretion. therefore

- ➤ To reduce estrogen, consume fiber and flax seeds.
- ➤ Use more cabbage family vegetables.
- ➤ Have exercise in your schedule.

Neuropeptide Y

Neuropeptide Y is produced in brain cells and the nervous system and increases when you are hungry or under pressure and stress and increases the desire to eat, obesity and accumulation of fat in the abdomen.

Recommendations to reduce neuropeptide Y secretion

➢ Consume enough protein.

➢ Do not starve for a long time.

➢ Do not forget to consume probiotic soluble fibers.

Glucagon-like peptide hormone 1

Glucagon-like peptide 1 hormone is secreted from the intestine after digestion. One of the causes of loss of appetite after weight loss surgery is the decrease in the production of this hormone.

Ways to increase the secretion of glucagon-like peptide 1 hormone

➢ Consume as much protein as you can, such as whey protein, yogurt and fish.

➢ Eat green vegetables such as spinach and kale.

➢ Include probiotic supplements and products in your meals.

Cholecystokinin hormone

Cholecystokinin hormone is secreted from intestinal cells. High amounts of this hormone reduce appetite and eating in both fat and thin people.

Hence, to increase cholecystokinin hormone

➢ Eat protein and healthy fats.

➢ Do not forget to consume fiber.

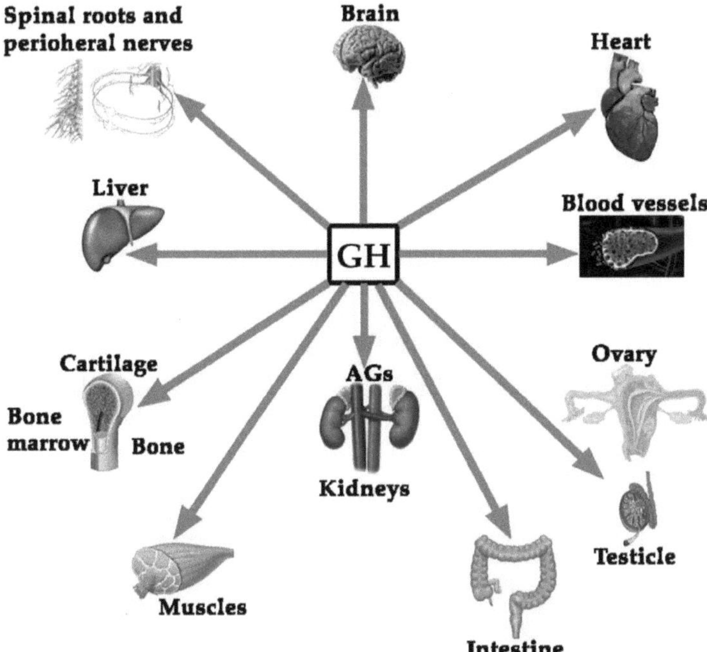

Figure 14. Growth Hormone (GH) and Cardiovascular System

Peptide YY hormone

Peptide YY hormone is another intestinal hormone that controls appetite and is secreted from the cells of the small intestine and large intestine. This hormone significantly reduces the amount of eating and the risk of obesity.

Therefore:

➢ Have a low carbohydrate diet, especially do not use processed foods. An increase in blood sugar destroys the effects of this hormone.

➢ Include both animal and vegetable protein as well as fiber in your meals.

"Hormones have a synergistic effect and are related to each other. Fortunately, diet modification and lifestyle changes have positive effects on hormones."

Types of female hormones; The role and effects of hormonal imbalance

Every woman deals with unique hormones. Understanding what types of female hormones are and how they play a role in your body is very important to maintain hormone health in a woman's life. Although the diagnosis of hormonal imbalance and how to treat it is the responsibility of the gynecologist, but if you have a good understanding of the role of female hormones, you will be more aware to recognize abnormal hormonal imbalance and deal with the natural decline of female hormones that occurs with age. In the following, we invite you to follow this article from doctor health magazine and learn more about the types of female hormones and their functions.

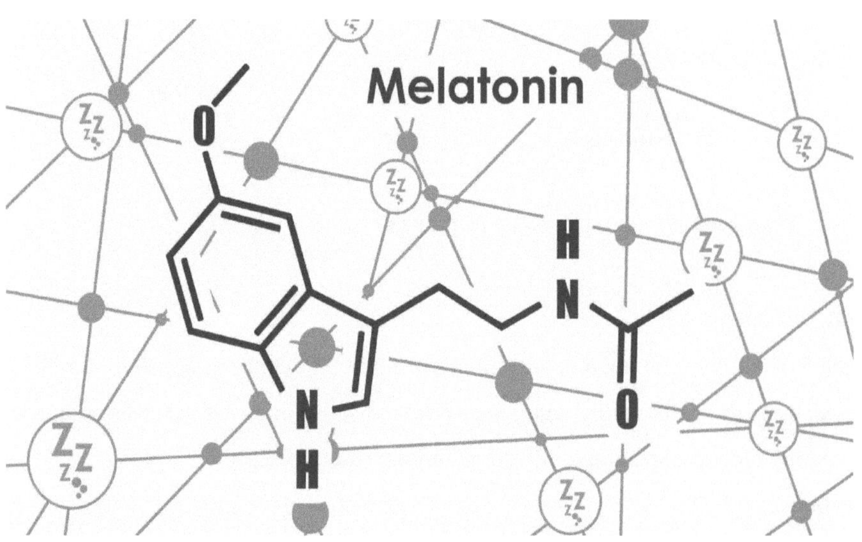

Figure 15. Anatomie des Menschen: Hormone - Hormone - Natur - Planet Wissen

Types of female hormones

Female hormones, which are also called sex steroids, play a very important role in reproduction and general health of women. Although the level of sex hormones changes over time, it changes more during periods such as menopause or menopause and even puberty than any other period. There are different types of female hormones that we will examine below

Estrogen

Estrogen is the most well-known type of female hormone. Most estrogen production occurs in the ovaries, however, estrogen can also be produced in the adrenal glands and adipose tissue (fat cells). There are four main estrogens in every woman:

> - Estrone is a weak estrogen that acts primarily as a precursor hormone.
> - Estradiol is the main estrogen responsible for many classic female characteristics.
> - Estriol is a weak estrogen that is mainly produced during pregnancy.
> - S-sterol is also a weak estrogen that is made during pregnancy and is only produced by the fetal liver.

Progesterone

Estrogen was first mentioned in 1934; Progesterone is a hormone found in both women and men. Progesterone stabilizes the menstrual cycle and prepares your body for a healthy pregnancy. This hormone can be produced in the ovaries, adrenal glands and placenta. Like other female hormones, progesterone levels are at their highest during ovulation and pregnancy.

Testosterone

Testosterone is primarily known as the male sex hormone. However, testosterone is also important for women's health. Healthy testosterone levels play a role in regulating menstruation, libido, bone strength, and muscle strength. Testosterone helps women have mental clarity of energy and helps you burn fat more effectively.

Adrenal glands and ovaries are responsible for the production of this hormone in women.

Different roles of female hormones over time

The types of female hormones during the period that are secreted in the body of every woman have a unique task.

Puberty

Females usually enter puberty between the ages of 8 and 13. Puberty occurs when the level of female hormones in the body increases rapidly. The pituitary gland produces luteinizing hormone and follicle-stimulating hormone, which increases the level of estrogen as well as progesterone and testosterone. Hormones associated with puberty cause several important physical changes:

- Increase in fat cells, especially in the hips and thighs;
- Breast growth;
- Growth of pubic, leg and armpit hair;
- Hip and hip widening;
- Maturation of ovaries, uterus and vagina;
- Beginning of the menstrual cycle;
- Growth spurt.

Menstruation

Menstruation usually starts at the age of 12. Female hormones regulate the menstrual cycle in three phases

Follicular phase

With the discharge of blood and uterine tissue through the vagina, the level of female hormones decreases. Follicle-stimulating hormone (FSH) and luteinizing hormone (LH) are produced, which stimulate the development of a new egg. As an egg is formed in the ovary, estrogen also increases.

Ovulation stage

During ovulation, the level of luteinizing hormone and estrogen reaches its peak and the dominant egg is released from the ovary. An egg can survive for up to a full day after release. Fertilization of the egg occurs only during this period.

Luteal phase

The egg enters the uterus through the fallopian tube. The ruptured follicle releases progesterone and thickens the lining of the uterus to prepare it to receive the fertilized egg. An unfertilized egg causes a decrease in estrogen and progesterone levels. This marks the beginning of the premenstrual week. Finally, the unfertilized egg and uterine wall are shed, marking the end of the current menstrual cycle and the beginning of the next period. A normal menstrual cycle repeats every 21 to 35 days; But irregular periods are quite common among women, especially for young women who are just starting their cycles and also for postmenopausal women who are nearing the end of their cycles.

Sexual desire

Testosterone, progesterone, and estrogen all play a role in sexual desire and arousal. Women's libido is usually highest right before the ovulation phase of the menstrual cycle. The use of hormonal contraceptives can lead to undesirable side effects such as decreased libido. Libido also decreases after menopause. Surgery to remove the adrenal glands or ovaries decreases female hormone production, possibly leading to decreased libido.

Pregnancy

The moment a fertilized egg implants in the uterine wall, the placenta begins to grow. The wall of the uterus thickens and is filled with important nutrients that support the fetus. Types of female hormones associated with pregnancy include: Relaxing, sterol, estriol, human chorionic gonadotropin (hCG), human placental lacto gen (second trimester). The increase in progesterone production in the first weeks of pregnancy tells the cervix to thicken and form a mucous plaque, which is very important to protect the fetus from infection. The rapid increase in estrogen and progesterone leads to nausea, vomiting and frequent urination, which are common symptoms of early pregnancy. After pregnancy ends, female hormones slowly return to lower levels than before pregnancy. Decreased hormone levels may cause postpartum depression. Breastfeeding can lower estrogen and may prevent ovulation. But breastfeeding alone is not considered an effective method of birth control.

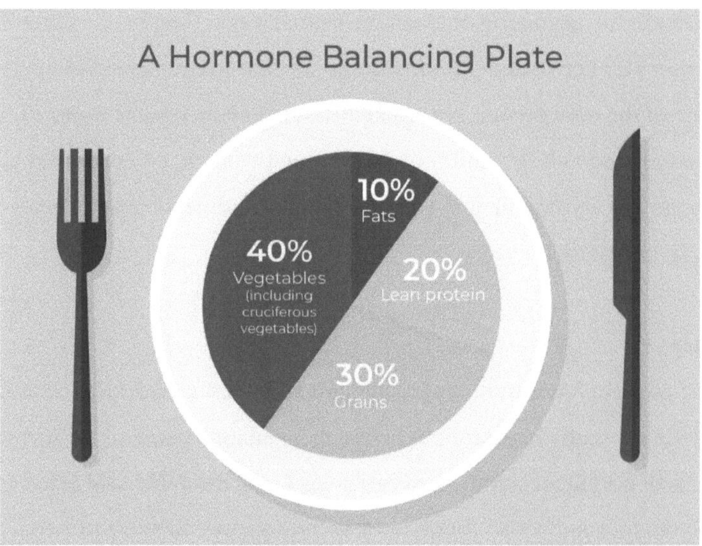

Figure 16. How Does Food Affect Your Hormones? | Marion Gluck Clinic

Pre-menopause and menopause

Perimenopause is the period leading up to menopause, which lasts on average between two and eight years. During pre-menopause, the production of various female hormones fluctuates and decreases. This hormonal fluctuation causes irregular periods or may stop them altogether. Menopause is defined as one year without a period. The average age for menopause is 51 years. Among the most important symptoms of pre-menopause and menopause, we can mention the following: insomnia, hot flashes, changes in mood, decreased libido and vaginal dryness. Low hormone levels during menopause often lead to women's health problems such as osteoporosis (thinning of the bones) and cardiovascular disease.

Causes of hormonal imbalance in women

Most women suffer from hormonal imbalance for various reasons. Common root causes of hormonal imbalances include: Certain medications, chronic stress, injury/trauma, Cushing's syndrome, adrenal problems, congenital adrenal hyperplasia, amenorrhea (absence of menstruation), appetite disorders, hypothyroidism or hyperthyroidism, hypogonadism, diabetes, hormone treatment, polycystic ovary syndrome (PCOS), cancer (especially of the ovaries or pituitary gland), chemotherapy, premenstrual syndrome (PMS), perimenopause or menopause, and miscarriage.

Normal levels of female hormones

A blood test determines the level of estrogen, progesterone and testosterone. These levels are:

➤ Normal estrogen levels are 15-350 pg./ml for an adult premenopausal woman and 10 pg./ml for an adult postmenopausal woman.

➤ The normal level of progesterone is 0.1 to 0.3 ng/ml at puberty to 290 ng/ml in the third trimester.

➤ The normal level of testosterone is 15 to 70 ng/dL.

Common symptoms of female hormone imbalance

Unfortunately, female hormones are not always in balance and sometimes they are in a state of imbalance. This change in hormonal schedule usually happens due to the following factors:

➤ Unexplained weight gains or loss;

➤ Fatigue;

➤ Sensitivity to cold or heat;

- ➤ Frequent bowel movements or frequent urination;
- ➤ Irregular heartbeat;
- ➤ Increased hunger or thirst;
- ➤ Breast tenderness;
- ➤ Depression;
- ➤ Flatulence;
- ➤ Decreased libido;
- ➤ Sterility;
- ➤ Hypothyroidism;
- ➤ Irregular periods;
- ➤ Excess hair on the face (called hirsutism);
- ➤ Excessive acne;
- ➤ Hair loss, hair thinning;
- ➤ Vaginal dryness;
- ➤ Vaginal atrophy;
- ➤ Night sweats;
- ➤ Pain during intercourse.

Natural methods to correct the imbalance of female hormones

Correcting hormonal balance goes beyond a one-sided attention to estrogen, testosterone and progesterone. Below we explore the many factors that can affect your hormone levels and overall health. Addressing all of these issues will not only help you balance your female hormones, but will also improve your quality of life:

- ➤ **Get enough sleep.** Try to sleep for 7 to 8 hours to give rest to different organs of the body, including the endocrine system. Sleep disorder affects hormones and often leads to obesity, diabetes and appetite problems.

- ➤ **Most technology devices emit blue light.** One hour before going to sleep, turn off devices that have screens; Because blue light can disrupt the natural circadian rhythm of your sleep.

➢ **Exercise is very important for general health.** Even short sessions of exercise can properly regulate hormone levels. Sometimes losing 10% of body fat can normalize menstrual periods.

You may have noticed that chronic stress can lead to hormonal imbalance. Find ways to reduce your daily stress. Even listening to music can reduce stress levels. Meditation, yoga, prayer and worship all help reduce stress levels.

Quit smoking. Obviously, tobacco is a known carcinogenic and addictive substance. Tobacco smoke also affects thyroid and pituitary gland function and can also increase levels of cortisol, a steroid hormone associated with stress. Too much alcohol also damages the liver, which is responsible for the production of several hormones. Therefore, it is wise to protect the liver and moderate alcohol consumption. If these lifestyle changes fail, you can turn to hormone therapy. Many look to biologic hormone therapy, which uses hormones that are chemically similar to those in your own body. This option offers a safer and more natural way to manage hormonal changes, especially after menopause.

A diet that balances female hormones

Eat healthy fats and plenty of fiber. Both of them play a role in the regulation of insulin hormone along with other types of female hormones. Fish are excellent sources of omega-3 fatty acids. Fatty fish helps prevent depression and anxiety. Omega-3 fatty acids also reduce inflammation, which many believe contributes to hormonal imbalances. Avoid sugar consumption.

Excess sugar leads to type 2 diabetes, obesity, metabolic disease, and more. Probiotics and adapt genic herbs promote hormone balance as well as immune system health and gut health. Hormonal overweight is a problem that women face more than men. If you are facing the problem of overweight without overeating or without giving up daily exercise, then your problem can be due to hormonal overweight. In order to better understand this issue, we suggest that you stay with us in the following article. Diagnosing hormonal overweight will sometimes be a challenging task for your doctor.

Because usually without having serious symptoms, hormone tests are hardly performed in medical centers.

However, there are signs through which you can be aware of this. In fact, the level of our hormones changes throughout life and this can cause symptoms in some people. For example, women in the short period before menopause or during their menopause are more likely to suffer from the problem of hormonal overweight.

In general, the following signs may be mentioned as warning signs to clarify whether your weight gain (as a woman) is caused by a hormonal overweight problem.

- Feeling unwell or bored;
- Increase hair growth;
- Being weak and low energy;
- Irregular menstrual periods.

Of course, in addition to examining the above symptoms, it is necessary to test the level of hyperactivity or hypothyroidism of women, and in addition to that, the two questions below should also be answered honestly by them. Of course, hormones are also fluctuating during the month, and if people are unlucky, this can lead to their hormonal weight gain. For example, during the second half of the menstrual cycle, women can experience a large decrease in the amount of progesterone hormone. This can cause problems related to hormonal overweight. Of course, it should be noted that not all hormones are involved in the problem of hormonal overweight, and only a few of them play a role in this matter.

The role of estrogen hormone in hormonal overweight

The dominant role of this hormone can lead to weight gain in women around the thigh and waist area.

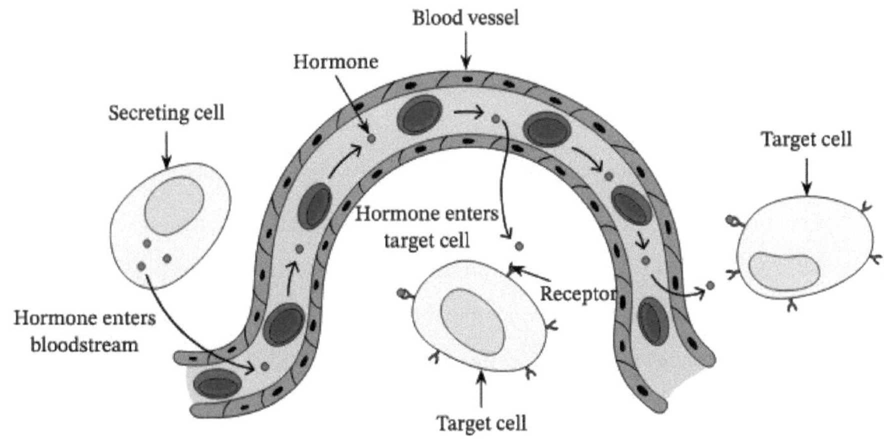

Figure 17. Lesson Explainer: Hormonal Control in Humans

The role of cortisol hormone in hormonal overweight

This hormone is associated with things like increased appetite, the desire to use sugary substances, and weight gain in the abdominal area. In addition, how to face stress and how to overcome stressful situations may also affect the type of reactivity of the adrenal cortical system to stress and the way fat is distributed.

The role of insulin hormone in hormonal overweight

This hormone controls our blood sugar levels. Accordingly, if we consume a lot of sugary substances, this can quickly lead to an increase in fat in the body. In fact, excessive absorption of sugar through consumption of processed and unhealthy foods or alcohol and even excessive consumption of fruits can lead to insulin-related problems. What can be called insulin resistance is a condition in which insulin is unable to effectively regulate blood glucose levels, and this can lead to an increase in sugar and then weight gain.

The role of leptin hormone in hormonal overweight

The hormone leptin plays a clever role in the body and warns us that we are full when we no longer need to eat. Also, this hormone plays a significant role in regulating and balancing the amount of energy. If we consume too much of unhealthy foods that contain sugar, our brain will show less sensitivity to leptin hormone. In this way, the feeling of satiety does not appear when necessary and this can ultimately lead to weight gain. Studies show that limited sleep can cause a change in activities related to body metabolism and the functioning of internal glands. Transformations that will bring shortcomings such as reducing the glucose limit, reducing insulin sensitivity, increasing leptin levels, and increasing cortisol levels. Changes that cause overall increase in appetite and weight.

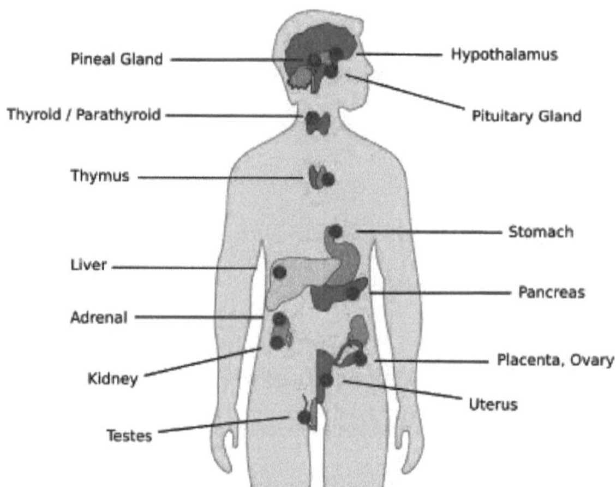

Figure 18. Hormone Antibodies, Kits, Proteins | www.antibodies-online.com

Chapter III

Genetic Diseases

Genetic diseases are diseases that are caused by genetic abnormalities in a person or are inherited from parents. Of course, genetic diseases are two separate types of gene mutations (such as thalassemia) or chromosomal disorders (such as Down's syndrome) are created.

Classification of genetic diseases

In fact, there are many factors that lead to the development of genetic diseases in a person, which can be detected in the laboratory. These factors are categorized as follows.

Predominant disorder

In this case, people inherit genetic disorders from their parents. In the dominant disorder, there is a 50% chance that one of the parents has a defective gene and will pass it on to the next generation.

Recessive disorder

In the recessive disorder, both parents have a defective gene and have passed it on to the next generation. Of course, the probability of this condition occurring in genetic diseases is 25%. Different types of hereditary genetic disorders can be divided into four categories: Monogenic hereditary disorders, multifactorial hereditary disorders, chromosomal abnormalities, and mitochondrial disorders.

Disorders related to gender

This type of disorder is always caused by genes on the (x) chromosome. Of course, it should be noted that genetic mutations often occur randomly or by some environmental factors.

All kinds of diseases, hereditary and genetic diseases

Down syndrome

Down syndrome is a genetic disorder that results from abnormalities during cell division and results in a complete or partial extra copy of chromosome 21. This extra genetic material causes developmental changes and physical characteristics. The disease varies in severity from person to person and causes lifelong intellectual disability and developmental delay. This syndrome is the most common genetic chromosomal disorder and cause of learning disability in children. It also commonly causes other medical abnormalities, including heart and gastrointestinal disorders.

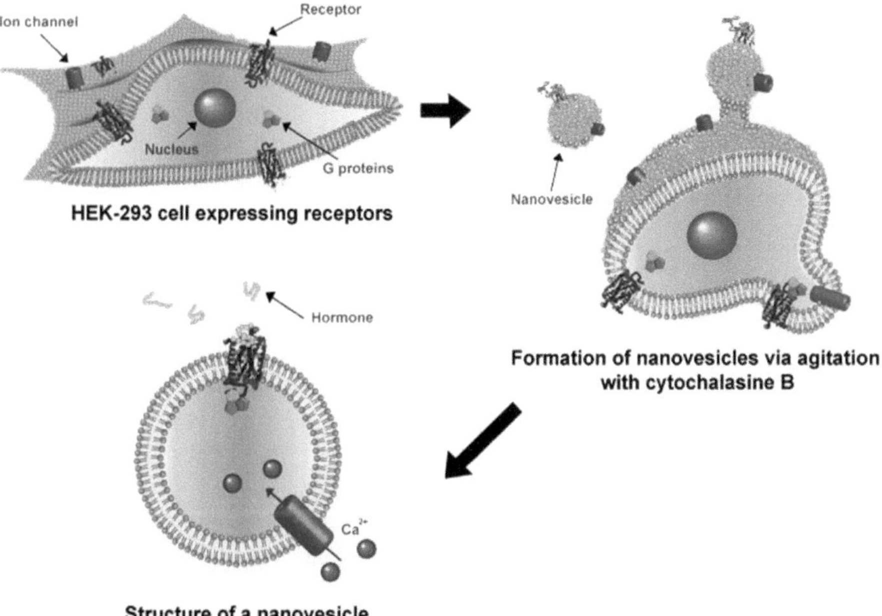

Figure 19. Peptide hormone sensors using human hormone receptor-carrying nanovesicles and graphene FETs

Signs

Affected children and adults have specific facial features.

Although not all sufferers have the same features, some common features include

> Flat face and small head;
> Short neck;
> Protruding tongue;
> The eyelids are abnormal;
> Unusual or small shaped ears;
> Muscle weakness;
> Wide and short hands with a palm crease;
> Relatively short fingers and small hands and feet;
> Excessive flexibility;
> There are small white spots on the colored part (iris) of the eye called Brushfield spots;
> Short.

Babies with Down syndrome may be average in size. But typically they grow slowly and are shorter than other children of the same age.

Causes of Down syndrome

Human cells normally contain 23 pairs of chromosomes. One chromosome from each pair is inherited from the father and the other from the mother. Down syndrome occurs when abnormal cell division occurs with chromosome 21. These cell division abnormalities result in partial or complete chromosome 21. This extra genetic material is responsible for the distinctive features and developmental problems of Down syndrome.

Any of three genetic conditions can cause Down syndrome

➢ **Trisomy 21.** About 95 percent of cases of this syndrome are caused by trisomy 21—a person has three copies of chromosome 21 in all cells instead of the usual two. It is caused by abnormal cell division during the development of the sperm cell or egg cell.

➢ **Mosaic Down syndrome.** In this rare form of Down syndrome, the person has only some cells with an extra copy of chromosome 21. This mosaic of normal and abnormal cells after fertilization is caused by the division of abnormal cells.

➢ **Translocation Down syndrome.** In this case, before or during the formation of a part of chromosome 21, it is connected to another chromosome. These children have two normal copies of chromosome 21, but they also have other genetic material from chromosome 21 that is attached to another chromosome.

Risk factors

Risk factors include the following

Some parents have a higher risk of having a child with Down syndrome.

➢ **Mother's age.** The probability of a woman giving birth to an affected child increases with age. Because larger eggs have a higher risk of improper chromosome division.

➢ **Carries the genetic transmission for Down syndrome.** Men and women can pass the genetic transmission of this disease to their children.

➢ **Having an affected child.** Parents who have one affected child and parents who themselves are displaced are at risk of having another child.

Complications

Affected individuals can have various complications, some of which become more prominent as they get older. These complications can include the following:

- ➤ **Heart defects.** About half of affected children are born with some form of congenital heart defect. These heart problems can be life-threatening and may require surgery in the early stages.

- ➤ **Defects of the digestive system.** Abnormalities of the digestive system occur in some children with this disease and may include abnormalities of the intestine, esophagus, trachea, and anus. The possibility of digestive problems such as gastrointestinal obstruction, heartburn (gastric reflux) or celiac disease may increase.

- ➤ **Immune disorders.** Due to abnormalities in the immune system, people with Down syndrome are at risk of developing autoimmune disorders, some types of cancer and infectious diseases such as pneumonia.

- ➤ **Sleep apnea.** Children and adults with Down syndrome are more at risk of obstructive sleep apnea due to the creation of soft tissues and skeletal changes that lead to obstruction of their airways.

- ➤ **Obesity.** People with Down syndrome are more likely to be obese compared to the general population.

- ➤ **Spine problems.** In some people with Down syndrome, the cervical vertebrae may not be positioned correctly. This position exposes them to serious spinal cord injury from excessive neck pressure.

- ➤ **Leukemia.** Affected young children have an increased risk of developing leukemia.

- ➤ **Dementia.** People with dementia are at higher risk.

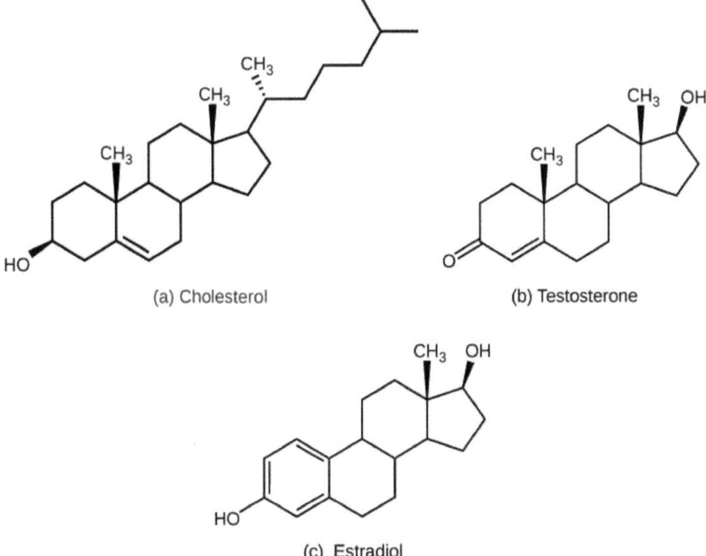

Figure 20. Types of Hormones – Concepts of Biology – 1st Canadian Edition

All kinds of diseases, hereditary and genetic diseases

Hemophilia

Hemophilia is a rare disorder in which the blood does not clot normally. And the reason is that the proteins related to blood clotting are either inactive or very low (clotting factors). In hemophilia, there is a risk of severe bleeding. Hemophilia is a genetic disorder. Treatment consists of regular replacement of clotting factors with blood products.

Signs

Symptoms of hemophilia vary depending on your clotting factor levels. If your clotting factor is mildly decreased, bleeding may occur only after surgery or injury. But if the deficiency is severe, spontaneous bleeding may also occur, which will threaten the person's health. Symptoms of bleeding in spontaneous hemophilia include the following:

- ➢ Unexplained and excessive bleeding from cuts or injuries or after surgery or dental work;
- ➢ Large or deep bruises;
- ➢ Unusual bleeding after vaccination;
- ➢ Pain, swelling or tightness in the joints;
- ➢ Blood in the urine or stool;
- ➢ Bleeding from the nose (nosebleeds).

Treatment of hemophilia

Hemophilia treatment for people who have a family history of this disease, it can be determined during pregnancy whether the fetus is affected by hemophilia or not. However, the test carries some risks to the fetus and is therefore performed at the discretion of the physician. In children and adults, blood tests can show clotting factor deficiency. Severe cases of hemophilia are usually diagnosed in the first year of life. Mild forms may not become apparent until adulthood. Some people first find out they have hemophilia after bleeding profusely during surgery.

Treatment

Several different types of clotting factors are associated with different types of hemophilia.

Main treatment for severe hemophilia

It consists of replacing the specific clotting factor required by the patient through the injection of blood products. Alternative clotting factor can be obtained from donated blood. similar products, recombinant clotting factors are produced in the laboratory and are not made from human blood.

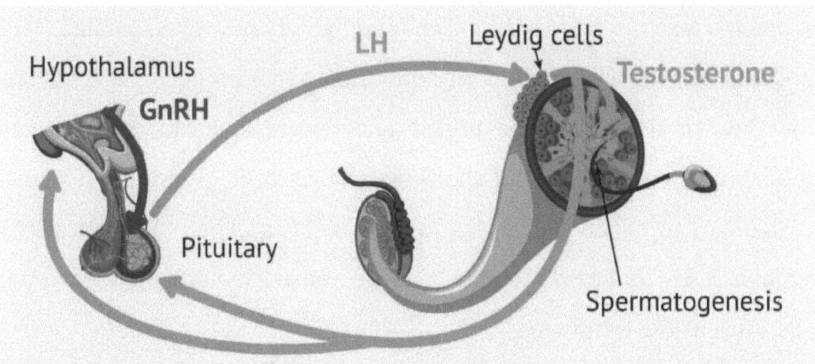

Figure 21. What are the functions of the LH hormone in the reproductive cycle?

Other treatments may include

> **Desmopressin.** This drug is effective in some types of mild hemophilia. This hormone can stimulate the body to release more clotting factor.

> **Anticoagulant drugs.** These drugs help prevent the clot from deteriorating.

> **Fibrin sealants.** These medications can be applied directly to wound sites to promote clotting and healing. Fibrin sealants are particularly useful in dentistry.

> **Physiotherapy.** If internal bleeding damages the joints, it may not have very specific symptoms. If the internal bleeding has caused severe injuries, surgery may be required.

All kinds of diseases, hereditary and genetic diseases, blood diseases

Favism disease

Favism disease or G6PD deficiency is a genetic abnormality that results in an inadequate amount of glucose-6-phosphate dehydrogenase (G6PD) in the blood. G6PD enzyme plays a role in regulating various biochemical reactions in the body. The G6PD enzyme is also responsible for keeping red blood cells healthy so they can function properly and have a normal lifespan. Without a sufficient amount of this enzyme, red blood cells break down prematurely. This initial destruction of red blood cells is known as hemolysis and can eventually lead to hemolytic anemia.

Hemolytic anemia occurs when red blood cells are rapidly destroyed and the rate of their destruction exceeds the rate of their replacement by new cells. As a result, it reduces the flow of oxygen to the organs and tissues and can cause fatigue, yellowing of the skin and eyes, and shortness of breath. In people with favism, hemolytic anemia can occur after eating a type of bean called "Fava beans" or certain legumes such as beans. It may also be caused by infection or certain medications, such as the following.

➢ Antimalarial is a type of medicine that is used to prevent and treat malaria.
➢ Sulfonamides are drugs that are used to treat various infections.
➢ Aspirin is a drug that is used to relieve fever, pain and swelling.
➢ Some non-steroidal anti-inflammatory drugs (NSAIDs).

Signs

Most people with favism usually do not experience any symptoms. However, some may develop symptoms when exposed to drugs, foods, or infections that cause premature destruction of red blood cells. Once the underlying cause is treated or resolved, the symptoms of G6PD deficiency usually disappear within a few weeks. Symptoms of G6PD deficiency (Favism disease) can include:

➢ Fast heartbeat;
➢ Shortness of breath;
➢ Dark or yellow-orange urine;
➢ Fever;
➢ Fatigue;
➢ Dizziness;
➢ Pallor;
➢ Jaundice or yellowing of the skin and whites of the eyes.

Risk factors

- ➤ **Gender.** The prevalence of this genetic disease is higher in men.
- ➤ **Race.** The prevalence of this disease is higher in some races such as African-Americans.
- ➤ **Geography.** This disease has a significant prevalence in the Middle East.
- ➤ **Family history.**

Diagnosis

- ➤ G6PD enzyme assay test;
- ➤ CBC test and blood reticulocyte count;
- ➤ Serum hemoglobin test.

All kinds of diseases, hereditary and genetic diseases

Chronic granulomatosis

Chronic granulomatosis (CGD) is a rare, inherited immunodeficiency that affects certain white blood cells. In patients with this disease, the function of the immune system is impaired and the body is exposed to chronic inflammation and frequent bacterial and fungal infections. Features of chronic granulomatosis usually appear in childhood or early childhood. However, milder forms may be diagnosed in the teenage years or even in adulthood. This disease is caused by gene changes (mutations) and is usually inherited by autosomal recessive or X-linked recessive method. People suffering from this disease must continuously use different antibiotics and be under the supervision of medical teams. The only treatment for this disease is allogeneic hematopoietic stem cell transplantation (HSCT).

Symptoms

In people with this disease, the immune system does not work properly and as a result, the body becomes vulnerable to certain types of bacteria and fungi. The characteristics of this disease usually appear in childhood or early childhood. However, milder forms may be diagnosed in the teenage years or even in adulthood.

Signs and symptoms vary but may include

> Frequent bacterial and fungal infections;

> Granuloma (areas of inflamed tissue), mostly in the digestive tract or genital tract;

> Occurrence of abscesses in lungs, liver, spleen, bones or skin;

> Swollen lymph nodes;

> Persistent diarrhea;

> Chronic runny nose.

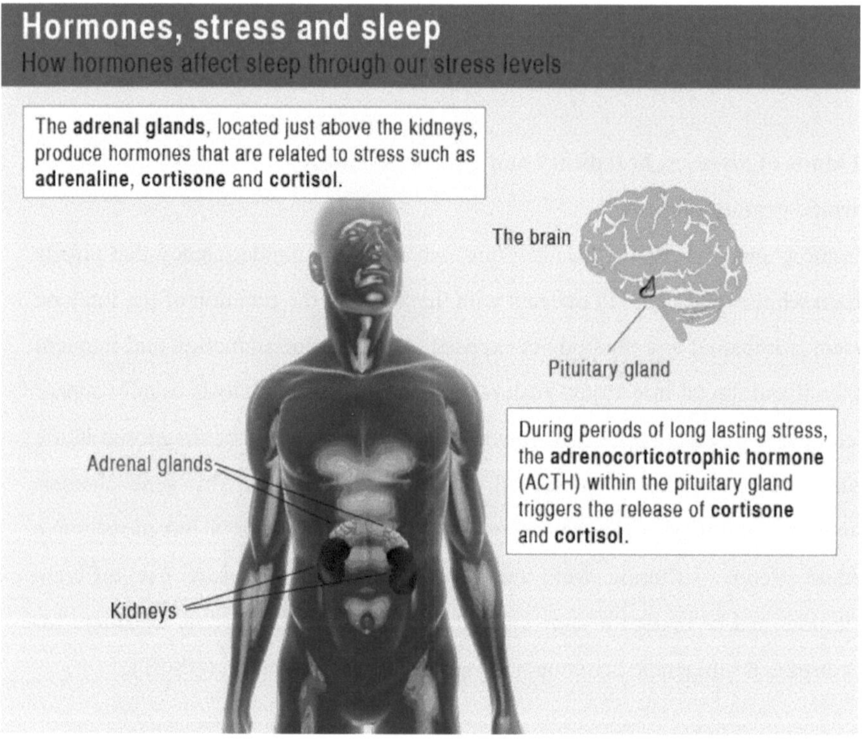

Figure 22.. Chemical messengers: how hormones help us sleep

Causes of granulomatosis

This disease is caused by a change (mutation) in one of five genes (CYBA, CYBB, NCF1, NCF2 or NCF4). Each gene encodes a different part (that subunit) of an enzyme called NADPH oxidase, which is essential for the body's immune system. One of the functions of this enzyme is to help make toxic substances that are used by the immune system to destroy bacteria and fungi. And it leads to the destruction of microbial agents before causing an infection. It may also play a role in regulating the activity of immune cells that help manage the inflammatory response. A decrease in these genes leads to a decrease in the level of NADPH oxidase, and in severe cases, no enzyme is produced. As a result, the body's immune system cannot function properly and the body is exposed to frequent infections and chronic inflammation.

All kinds of diseases, hereditary and genetic diseases

Alkaptonuria

Alkaptonuria is a rare hereditary disease. This disease occurs when the body cannot produce enough of an enzyme called homogenous dioxygenase (HGD). The task of this enzyme is to break down an excretory and toxic substance called homo genetic acid. Homo genic acid accumulates in the body when not enough HGD is produced. In fact, this is a rare disease. Accumulation of homogenous acid causes bones and cartilage to break down and become brittle. This typically leads to arthritis, especially in the spine and large joints.

Alkaptonor symptoms

In people suffering from alkaptonuria, the urine is dark and when exposed to air, its color becomes dark brown or black. Dark spots on a child's diaper are one of the first signs of this disease. There are no other symptoms in childhood. The symptoms become more obvious with age. At the age of 20 to 30, early arthritis symptoms may appear. For example, stiffness or chronic pain may be felt in the lower back or large joints. Other symptoms of alkaptonuria

➢ Dark spots in the whites of the eyes;

➢ Thick and dark cartilage in the ear;

➢ Discoloration and blue spots on the skin, especially in the sweat glands;

➢ Sweat turns dark;

➢ Kidney stone;

➢ Prostate stones;

➢ Arthritis (especially hip and knee joints).

Alkaptonuria can also lead to heart problems.

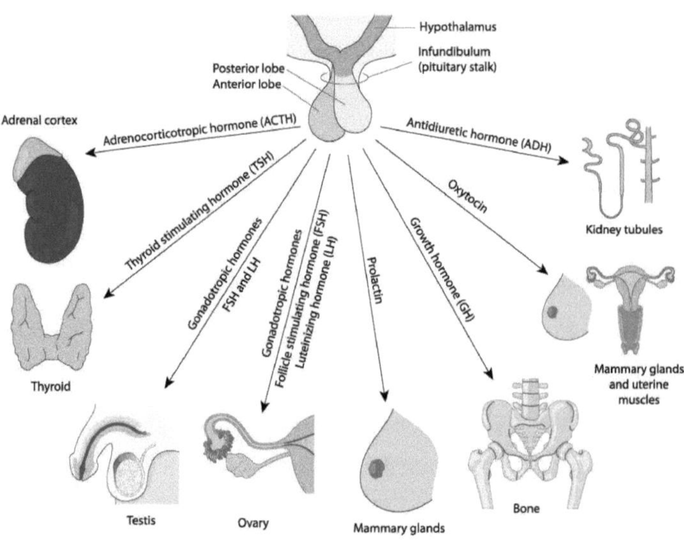

Figure 23. Hormone Testing | London Fertility Centre

Homo genic acid build-up causes heart valves to harden and this can prevent them from closing properly and lead to aortic and mitral valve disorders. In severe cases, heart valve replacement may be necessary. It also causes blood vessels to harden, which raises blood pressure.

Causes of infection

The causes of alkaptonuria occur as a result of genetic mutations in the gene coding for the HGD enzyme. This disease is an autosomal recessive disease and both parents of the patient have the corresponding gene. According to some researches, people who have a first-degree relative with depression are two to three times more at risk of developing depression than normal people.

This can be caused by hereditary depression or genetic depression. However, some people who suffer from depression do not have a family history of this mental disorder.

What is depression and what are its types?

While feelings of sadness, general boredom or lethargy are normal, depression causes long-term feelings of sadness, emptiness, or hopelessness. This disease is accompanied by a loss of interest in activities that you once enjoyed. These feelings can interfere with your ability to perform everyday activities. Some of the symptoms of depression include:

- Decreased energy and fatigue;
- Sleeping too little or too much;
- Difficulty concentrating;
- Change in weight and change in appetite;
- Unexplained pains;
- Anxiety;
- Irritability;
- Feelings of guilt, worthlessness or helplessness;
- Restlessness or difficulty sitting still;
- Suicidal thoughts or behaviors.

Types of depression include clinical depression, bipolar depression, postpartum depression, and seasonal depression. Among all these, some believe that hereditary depression can also be investigated as a separate type. Also, this type of depression may be effective in creating other types.

Is depression hereditary?

Watching a family member or relative suffer from depression can be a painful experience. If one of your family members is suffering from depression, the probability of developing it is 5 times higher. After several studies that observed this pattern in families, it became clear that this disease can be hereditary and has a critical genetic component. Researchers believe that there is a genetic component to depression and are still researching to prove it. But now there is no clear heritability pattern for depression. Studies show that changes in many genes increase the risk of developing depression.

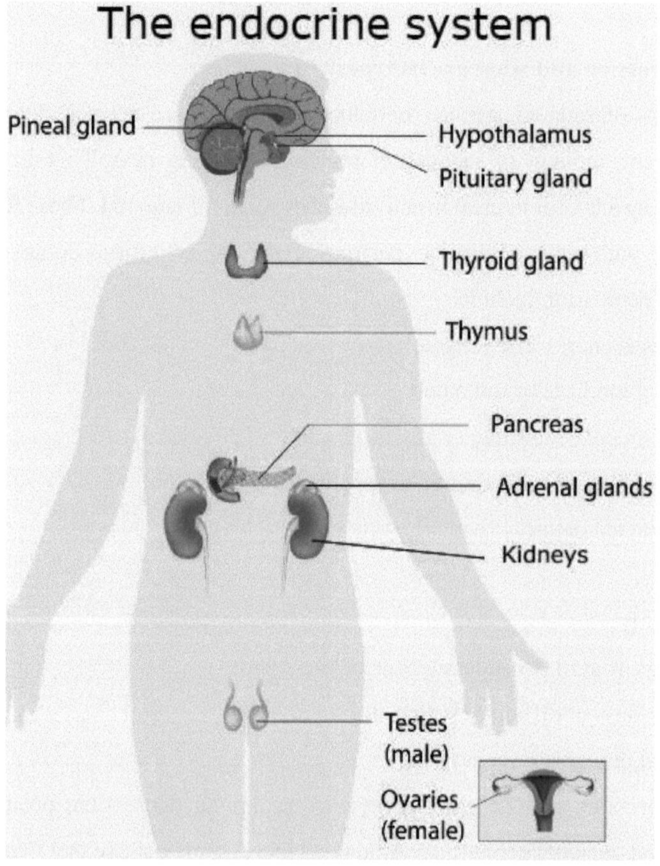

Figure 24. Endocrine glands and their hormones | healthdirect

Genes thought to be associated with depression have different functions in the brain. Some of them may control the production, transport and activity of chemicals called neurotransmitters. These transmitters send chemical signals and allow nerve cells (neurons) to communicate with each other.

Other genes that may affect the risk of depression are involved in the growth, maturation and maintenance of neurons. They also affect the ability of connections between neurons to change and adapt over time. For example, it is hypothesized that genes associated with low levels of the neurotransmitters serotonin, norepinephrine, and dopamine can lead to depression.

These neurotransmitters are responsible for regulating mood, sleep and appetite. Genetics may indicate the risk of developing depression, but it does not always determine whether a person will develop the disorder. If you are told that you have a gene for depression, you may worry that this disease will come to you in the future. However, having a genetic predisposition to a disease does not always mean you will get it. Rather, it means that you may be more susceptible to it than a person who does not have the same genetic structure.

So how much does genetics play a role in depression?

As far as researchers know, it is the interplay of genes and other factors such as the environment that determine whether a person develops depression. Some studies have shown that the probability of depression in a person who has one of his first-degree relatives is 5 times higher than other people who did not have depression in their family. Because genes play a role in the potential risk of many diseases, including depression. Heredity is a complex interplay of many factors and not just individual genes. When studying depression or other health conditions, researchers often look for changes in genes called variants.

These changes are classified based on the effect on genes. Eye color is an example of the effect of different types on genes. Changes in certain genes that affect melanin production, as well as several other genes, determine your eye color. You inherit a unique combination of genes from your parents. Families can often predict a child's eye color by looking at parents and other close relatives. But all kinds of genes can act unexpectedly. For example, parents with blue eyes may have a child with brown eyes. As a result, genetics plays a role in depression, but it is not the only main factor.

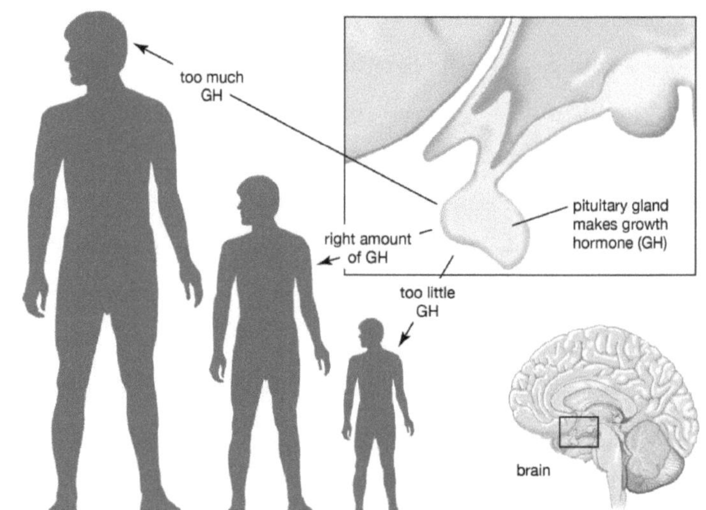

Figure 25. Growth hormone, Definition, Function, Deficiency, & Excess

Is depression transmitted from parents to children?

People with depression may worry about passing it on to their children. While there may be a genetic component to depression, genetics is not the only determining factor and other factors play a role in developing the disease.

A child with a depressed parent may have a genetic predisposition, but will not necessarily become depressed. Other factors are also involved, including environmental factors or triggers. On the other hand, a child who does not have a family member with depression and is not genetically predisposed to this disease may develop depression if exposed to a stimulating event such as experiencing a trauma.

In any case, even if depression does not run in your family, all parents should take the symptoms of depression seriously in children and adolescents.

Can hereditary depression be treated?

Yes, the treatment of hereditary depression is almost the same as the treatment of other depressions. In order to make sure of this issue, a research was done at Northwestern University.

In this experiment, some mice were genetically bred for depression. Then these mice received methods equivalent to psychotherapy and their depression improved. After the depressed mice were treated, some of their blood biomarkers for depression changed to non-depressed levels.

What are the non-genetic causes of depression?

Genetics is one of several potential causes of depression. Knowing the possible causes can help you better understand depression. But you must remember that depression can also occur in the absence of a clear cause, and it is difficult to accurately diagnose it. Other known factors that contribute to depression and other mental health conditions include:

- **Brain chemistry:** People with depression sometimes have lower levels of neurotransmitters. These transporters may be ineffective or poorly functioning.
- **Changes in brain structure:** The brains of people with depression may differ physically and structurally from the brains of people who are not depressed.
- **Hormones:** Conditions such as pregnancy, thyroid disorders and menopause can affect the level of hormones. Low or high levels of hormones can cause symptoms of depression, especially in people who are genetically predisposed. In addition to these, trauma and inappropriate environmental conditions can also cause depression.

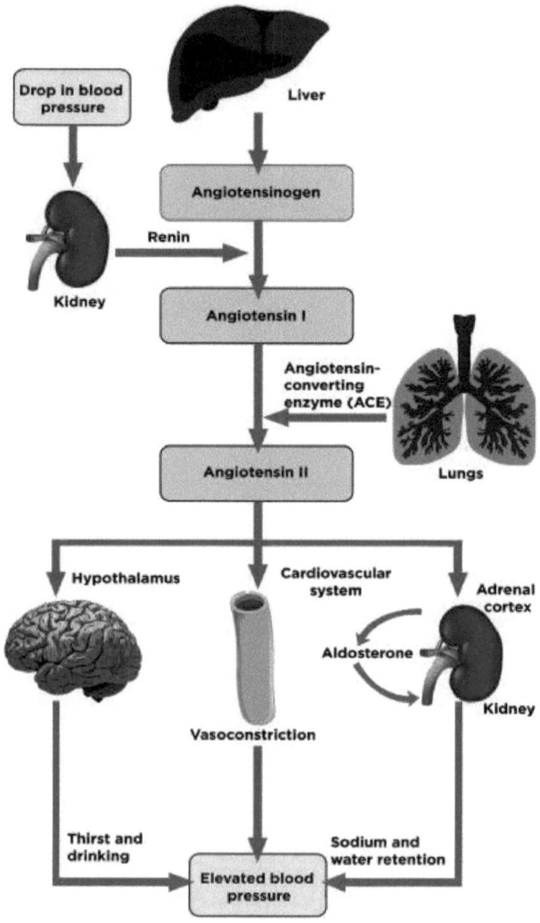

Figure 26. Liver Hormones - ScienceDirect

Do not forget to consult a specialist.

Depression is a disease that anyone can suffer from. However, how this disease is treated and managed depends on the type of treatment and your cooperation. At Doctor, we have created the best conditions for accessing online appointments so that you can quickly talk to a specialist for your mental and emotional challenges. If you are struggling with mental problems, you can get an appointment from the list of psychologists.

Is depression transmitted from parents to children?

Depression can be hereditary, but it is not definitely passed from parent to child. Other conditions such as environmental conditions also affect the disease.

Is it possible to prevent the hereditary transmission of depression?

Depression is often caused by a chemical imbalance in the brain, so there is no surefire way to prevent it. Hereditary depression can be controlled and treated only by considering the symptoms and their follow-up. Hereditary diseases or genetic disorders refer to a set of diseases that are caused by changes in the genetic material of a person and are passed from one generation to another. In fact, abnormality and genetic diseases occur as a result of mutations or changes in the body's chromosomes.

In ancient times, the diagnosis of genetic diseases was unpredictable, but today, modern medicine is able to identify genetic disorders and diseases to a large extent, and this can give us hope for the treatment of these diseases in the future.

What is a genetic disease?

A genetic disease occurs when a mutation or abnormality affects a person's genes and causes him to develop a specific disease. More than half of our genes come from our biological parents. Genetic mutations may pass from one or both parents to the child. Sometimes the symptoms of genetic disorders are caused by inheritance in a person's chromosomes, and sometimes genetic mutations are activated by chance or due to exposure to certain conditions by environmental factors. The creation of genetic mutations in the sequence and arrangement of DNA causes hereditary diseases.

All types of genetic disorders

Hereditary diseases and genetic disorders have different types. In the following, you can learn more about the types of hereditary diseases.

Chapter IV

Monogenetic hereditary disease

Monogenic or monogenic hereditary diseases occur when genetic changes occur on the DNA sequence of a single gene. Single-gene disorders are usually autosomal dominant (through one parent), autosomal recessive (through both parents), and are caused by the X chromosome. Diseases such as cystic fibrosis, thalassemia, sickle cell anemia, Marfan syndrome, Huntington's disease, and hemochromatosis are among the most common single-gene hereditary diseases.

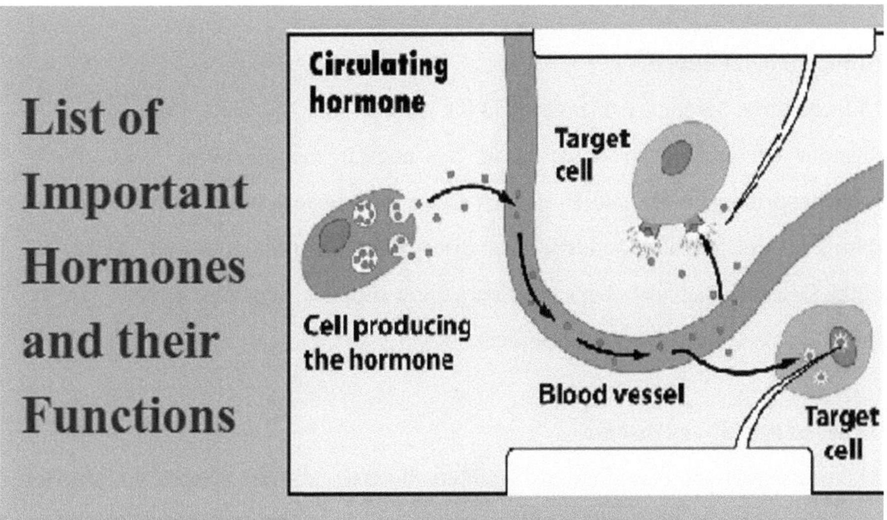

Figure 27. Insulin and Growth Hormone Balance: Implications for Obesity: Trends in Endocrinology & Metabolism

Multifactorial hereditary disease

Environmental and hereditary factors are involved in the occurrence of multifactorial or polygenic hereditary diseases. Diseases such as heart disease, high blood pressure, Alzheimer's, arthritis, diabetes, cancer and obesity are in the category of multifactorial hereditary diseases.

Chromosomal abnormalities

This type of genetic disorder is related to the number and structure of chromosomes. In fact, chromosomal abnormalities usually occur due to problems related to cell division. Diseases such as Down's syndrome, Turner's syndrome, Klinefelter's syndrome and crying cat syndrome are among the most common chromosomal abnormalities. Chromosome abnormalities are one of the most important causes of hereditary diseases.

Mitochondrial disorders

Mitochondrial hereditary disorder is in the last category of genetic disorders. This disorder occurs due to mutation of non-nuclear mitochondrial DNA. Each mitochondrion contains 5 to 10 circular DNA. Oocyte cells preserve mitochondria during fertilization and therefore these diseases are inherited only from mother to child. Diseases such as Leber's hereditary optic atrophy, myoclonic epilepsy are in the category of mitochondrial disorders.

Types of hereditary diseases

Many diseases are classified as hereditary diseases and are caused by genetic disorders in the body. In the following, you can learn about the most common hereditary diseases.

Down syndrome

Down syndrome is one of the most common hereditary diseases and the most well-known chromosomal disorder caused by the presence of 3 copies of chromosome number 21. People with Down syndrome have special mental and physical symptoms. There is no cure for this disease to date, and statistics show that one out of every 700 people has this disorder.

Hemophilia

Another common hereditary disease is hemophilia, which is caused by a defect in the blood coagulation system. This disease is more common in men and the symptoms of the disease vary from person to person according to the severity of the disease. There is no definitive treatment for this disease, and to control it, blood clot preservation drugs, tissue adhesives, and regular DDAVP injections are used. Hemophilia is a hereditary disease caused by a blood coagulation defect.

Sickle cell anemia

A genetic disease and anemia disorder that causes abnormal appearance of hemoglobin. In this disease, hemoglobin molecules are clustered together and therefore cannot easily pass through the capillaries. For the treatment of this disease, intravenous fluid injection, treatment of underlying infections, blood transfusion and bone marrow transplantation are used.

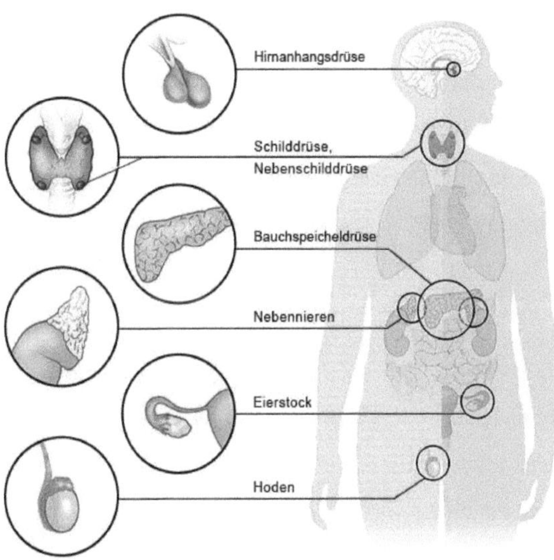

Figure 28. Welche Aufgaben haben die Hormone?

Celiac disease

Celiac disease is a common gastrointestinal disease that causes sensitivity to protein in wheat and barley. People with celiac disease should not use gluten-containing products because the body's immune system attacks the intestinal cells. These people should use gluten-free diets to prevent symptoms.

Homocystinuria

This genetic disorder causes a disturbance in the digestion of some amino acids in a person. In fact, people suffering from this disease do not have the ability to digest the amino acid methionine, and therefore they have problems after consuming these proteins. There is no cure for this disease, but taking high doses of vitamin B6 can help reduce the symptoms of the disease.

Crohn's disease

A type of genetic disease related to the intestine that causes inflammation in the digestive system. This painful disease, which is also called ileitis or enteritis, can cause problems and inflammation in the intestine from the mouth to the anus. Crohn's disease does not have a definitive cure, but the use of anti-inflammatory drugs, cortisone or steroids and the use of antibiotics can help reduce the symptoms of the disease. On the other hand, in some cases, it is necessary to undergo surgery for treatment.

Cystic fibrosis

Hereditary cystic fibrosis causes severe damage to the lungs, digestive system, and vital organs and affects mucus cells, sweat, and digestive juices. For the treatment of cystic fibrosis, drugs such as antibiotics, expectorant drugs, and non-steroidal anti-inflammatory drugs are usually used. In some cases, it is necessary for a person to undergo surgery for treatment.

Birth defects

Many birth defects such as cleft lip, neural tube defects, and heart problems are hereditary diseases at birth that are caused by genetic factors or excessive alcohol use in the fetus. Surgical methods can be used to treat some birth defects. One of the most obvious birth defects is cleft lip.

Alzheimer's disease

Alzheimer's is a type of genetic disorder that causes loss of memory and thinking power and makes a person unable to perform simple daily tasks. This disease starts slowly and gradually its severity will increase.

Hypothyroidism

This hereditary disease, which usually occurs in women over 60 years of age, occurs when the thyroid hormone is not secreted enough in the body and causes diseases such as obesity, joint pain, and heart disease. Hypothyroidism can be treated with pills and medications, as well as lifestyle changes.

MS disease

MS is another type of genetic disease that affects the brain and spinal cord and causes a person to lose balance, vision and senses. In this autoimmune disease, the body's immune system attacks the brain and spinal cord, which control the central nervous system, and causes paralysis and organ failure.

To treat MS, it is necessary to change your lifestyle and use a healthy diet and relaxation techniques. Doing meditation, yoga and traditional medicine are also effective for treating MS. The use of oral drugs and bone marrow stem cell transplantation are also among the most common methods of treating this disease.

Color blind

Color blindness is a genetic disease related to the X chromosome that causes a person not to recognize certain colors. In fact, people with color blindness see certain colors as gray and black. Special glasses, lenses or gene therapy can be used to treat color blindness.

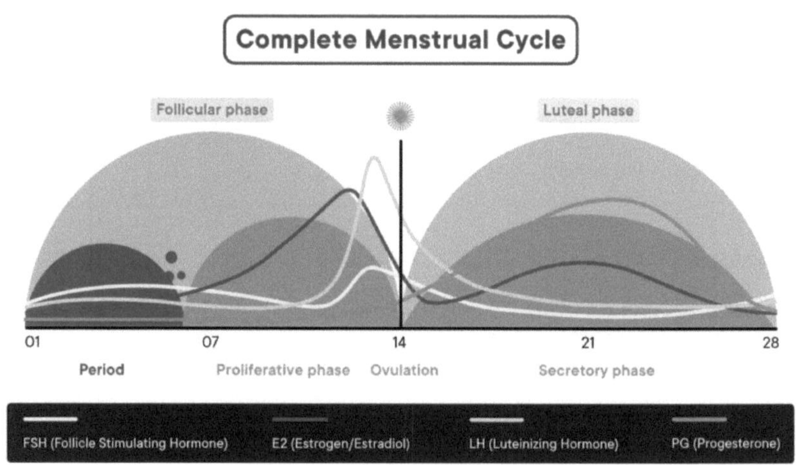

Figure 29. The Menstrual Cycle: Phases of Your Cycle

Leprosy disease

A type of genetic disease that causes the amount of pigment in the skin, hair and eyes to be zero, and therefore the color of the hair and skin of these people is completely white. Pale people usually have gray, blue or light hazel eyes. Leprosy is a type of genetic disease that causes loss of skin and hair pigments in the body.

Thalassemia

In this disease, a person's body does not produce enough hemoglobin, and therefore, not enough oxygen reaches the body's organs. People with thalassemia have different symptoms according to the severity of the disease and are known as minor and major. These people should use blood transfusions or supplement pills for treatment according to the severity of the disease.

Symptoms of genetic disorders and hereditary diseases

Genetic disorders have a very wide range, and depending on the type of disorder, it can lead to different symptoms in the body. But usually, these diseases appear in specific ways, which sometimes cause appearance abnormalities and sometimes cause specific diseases. Some of the most common symptoms of genetic disorders and hereditary diseases are mentioned below.

- Behavioral disorders;
- Breathing problems;
- Cognitive defects;
- Developmental delays;
- Digestive problems;
- Organ abnormalities;
- Movement disorders;
- Nervous problems;
- Poor growth;
- Reduced vision;
- Hearing loss.

Cause of hereditary disease

To understand the cause of hereditary disease and genetic disorders, it is better to first explain a little about how genes and DNA work. The DNA contained in the genes of our body is responsible for making proteins in the body. These proteins initiate complex cellular interactions and help our bodies stay healthy. Now, if a mutation occurs, the protein-making instructions of the genes will be affected and the protein-making process will face problems. Usually, environmental factors such as exposure to chemicals, exposure to harmful radiation, smoking, and exposure to ultraviolet rays are responsible for causing genetic mutations. In the following, several causes of abnormalities in hereditary diseases are mentioned.

- Abnormalities in chromosomes;
- Abnormality in a particular gene;

➢ Occurrence of abnormality due to environmental factors;

➢ Anomaly due to the presence of teratogens.

Hereditary disease treatment method

Most genetic disorders and hereditary diseases do not have specific treatment, and some of them have treatments that prevent the progression of the disease and the occurrence of symptoms to some extent. Usually, the type of treatment is considered according to the type of disease and its severity. However, early diagnosis of hereditary diseases is the best way to prevent the progress and control of the disease.

➢ In many cases, drugs and chemotherapy methods are used to control symptoms and treat hereditary diseases.

➢ Compliance with diets and lifestyle changes can help reduce the symptoms of genetic disorders to a great extent.

➢ In many cases, it is necessary for a person to undergo surgery to treat genetic disorders and repair abnormal body structure or to treat complications.

➢ Organ transplantation and replacing a healthy organ with a damaged one is another method of treating genetic diseases.

Methods of diagnosing genetic disorders

If you have a family history of a genetic disorder, doing genetic tests can show what diseases you have or whether you are susceptible to a certain genetic disease or not. In many cases, carrying a genetic mutation does not mean that a person will get that disease, but being in certain conditions and not protecting health can lead to the appearance of symptoms of the disease in a person.

➢ To diagnose genetic disorders, it is usually necessary for you and your partner to take blood tests before pregnancy to make sure that you have the potential to develop a certain genetic disorder.

➢ Screening tests are performed before birth to determine the percentage of the fetus suffering from chromosomal diseases.

➢ Prenatal diagnosis tests are performed in order to check genetic disorders in the fetus and are considered the best way to diagnose hereditary and genetic diseases.

➢ Newborn screening is done to detect genetic disorders early in life. Screening tests are used to diagnose hereditary diseases in babies.

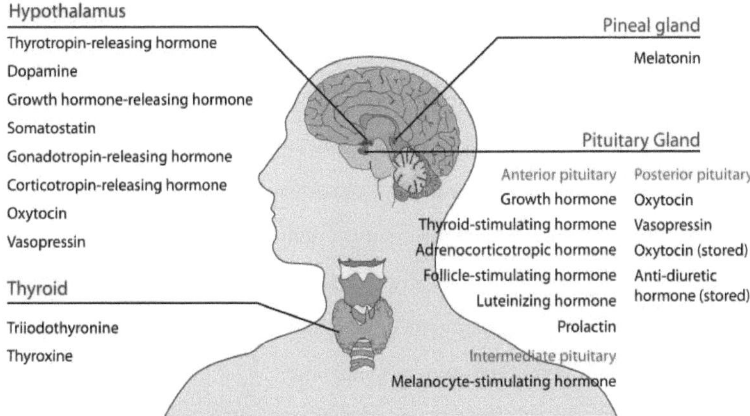

Figure 30. What is the Difference Between Direct and Indirect Hormone Action - Pediaa.Com

Method of preventing hereditary diseases

There is usually no specific way to prevent hereditary diseases. However, early diagnosis of genetic diseases as well as not being exposed to factors that cause the disease to worsen can be effective in preventing it.

➢ In order to prevent the transmission of hereditary diseases to the next generation, men and women should perform the necessary genetic tests before trying to get pregnant.

➢ The use of drugs, drugs, alcohol and unhealthy lifestyle can increase the risk of genetic diseases.

➤ To prevent the transmission of hereditary diseases, it is sometimes necessary to create an embryo by artificial insemination and to be examined for genetic disorders.

Genetic mutations and their role

Usually, genetic tests seek to find specific hereditary changes (mutations) in chromosomes, genes or proteins of a person. Genetic mutations can be harmful, beneficial or neutral to health. Harmful mutations increase the chance of developing diseases such as cancer. In general, it is said that hereditary mutations play an important role in 5-10% of all cancers. Sometimes cancers appear in a "Familial" way, even if the cause is not a hereditary mutation. For example, the common lifestyle (for example, using tobacco) is an important factor in the occurrence of similar cancers in people of the same family. Although specific patterns such as the type and age of cancer onset, the diagnosis of co-morbidities other than cancer may suggest the existence of a hereditary cancer syndrome.

What is a cancer test?

Many genetic mutations are known to cause hereditary cancers. In this regard, genetic tests can confirm the presence or absence of hereditary conditions for diagnosed cancer. Also, with the help of genetic tests, members of a family without having an obvious disease can be examined in terms of being carriers for specific hereditary mutations. Inherited genetic mutations increase a person's risk of cancer through different mechanisms (based on gene function). For example, mutations in genes that control cell growth and DNA repair increase the risk of developing cancer. All cancers begin with a genetic change, but only 10% of cancers are completely inherited.

Types of hereditary cancers

➢ Breast Cancer;

➢ Colon Cancer;

➢ Gastric cancer;

➢ Uterus cancer;

➢ Skin Cancer;

➢ Ovarian cancer;

➢ Pancreatic cancer;

➢ Prostate Cancer.

There are cancers that are included in the list of hereditary cancers.

Genetic testing for cancer

Genetic testing can be a useful option if there is any reason you or if you know someone who may be at risk for hereditary cancers. These genetic tests are used to diagnose cancer that can be inherited from one generation to another.

Does a person who inherits a cancer-predisposing mutation always get cancer?

Even if there is a mutation predisposing to cancer in the family, it does not necessarily mean that the person carrying the mutation will get cancer. Various factors affect the occurrence of cancer in people carrying mutations. One of these factors is the inheritance pattern of cancer. To better understand how cancer is inherited, it should be considered that each person has two copies of each gene, each of which he inherited from his two parents. Most of the mutations responsible for hereditary cancer are inherited in two ways:

➢ Autosomal dominant;

➢ Autosomal recessive.

Autosomal dominant inheritance

In autosomal dominant inheritance, the presence of only one copy of the mutated gene increases the chance of developing cancer. In this case, the individual's parents may show the effects of the mutated gene or just carry the mutated gene.

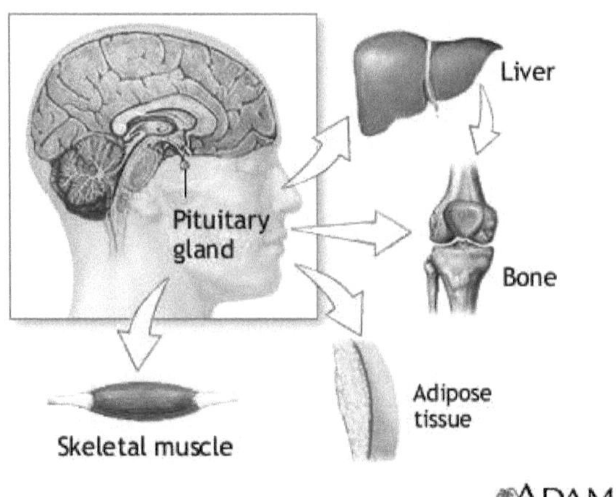

Figure 31. Growth hormone stimulation test - series—Normal anatomy: MedlinePlus Medical Encyclopedia

Autosomal recessive inheritance

In the case of autosomal recessive inheritance, a person has an increased risk of developing cancer only if they have inherited both copies of the mutated gene from their parents. In this case, parents who carry a mutated copy and a healthy copy of the relevant gene usually do not face an increased risk of cancer.

X-linked inheritance

The third form of inheritance of cancer predisposing gene is X-linked inheritance. While men have only one copy of the X chromosome, which is inherited from their mother, women have two copies of the X chromosome, each inherited from one of their parents. A woman with a recessive cancer-predisposing mutation on one of her X chromosomes does not face an increased risk of cancer as a carrier. However, her son, who inherited the mutated version of the gene, faces this increased risk. However, even if a person carries a mutated version of the desired gene with dominant inheritance; or has inherited both copies of the mutated gene with recessive inheritance; Or if a man's X chromosome carries a mutated version with recessive inheritance, they will not necessarily get cancer. Some mutations have "Incomplete penetrance" meaning that only some people show the effects of the mutation. Some mutations also have "Variable expression" in the sense that the severity of symptoms varies from person to person.

The role of heredity in the development of breast cancer
Usually 5-10% of all cancers are hereditary. This point includes all types of cancer, including breast cancer. In general, finding such cases by geneticists is not only very important in determining the level of risk in affected people, but it can also identify high-risk family members and prevent the transmission of known mutations to the next generations and, as a result, their disease. One of these diseases is hereditary breast cancer.

Breast cancer is very important as a common disease among women. It is emphasized once again that all cancers are genetic, that is, they are caused by changes in genes, but only about 5-10% of them are hereditary and are only passed on to children, and most of them are not passed on to children. Therefore, about 90-95% of cancers are not hereditary and cannot be passed on to children. These types of cancer are caused by other factors such as environmental factors and so on.

A percentage of cancers are familial, which means that the close family of the affected person is slightly more likely to get cancer than normal people in the society. Therefore, the difference in meaning of the words "Genetic", "Hereditary" and "Familial" should be paid attention to.

Hereditary breast cancer

Finding genetic material among breast cancer patients is very important. Many patients worry about their children getting the same disease, regardless of whether they have the disease themselves. In general, any woman up to the age of 80 may get breast cancer with a probability of about 80%. Today, many risk factors such as reduced physical activity, weight gain, use of steroid drugs, lack of breastfeeding, and use of carcinogens such as alcohol and smoking increase the risk of breast cancer.

Another risk factor can be seen in the hereditary type of this disease. As mentioned earlier, each gene, which is usually in pairs, is responsible for the inheritance of a trait. This mutation usually happens either for the first time when the cell that creates the embryo is formed at the time of conception, or it is passed on to the child from the sex cells of the father or mother. Therefore, all body cells contain this mutation. For this reason, all body cells can be used to check it. From a practical point of view, the most convenient cells are blood lymphocytes, which are obtained using a simple blood draw. Lymphocytes are a type of white blood cell.

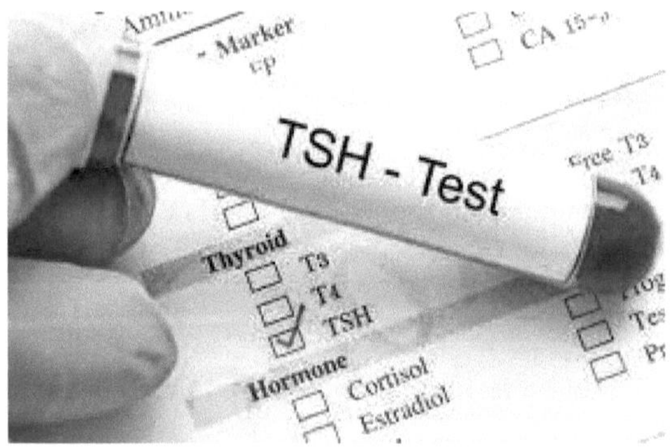

Figure 32. Hormone Disorders

Factors affecting hereditary breast cancer

The following are conditions that may indicate hereditary breast cancer. As it was said, these cases only raise the possibility of infection and it is necessary to get guidance from genetic counseling in these cases and perform additional tests if necessary:

❖ The disease is diagnosed at a younger age than its common age. Usually, this disease occurs in women over 45 years old, so if a person younger than this age is diagnosed with the disease, they should see a genetic counselor.

❖ More than one member of the family suffering from the same cancer (for example, breast cancer) or related cancer (for example, ovarian cancer), of course, if there is any type of cancer among the family members, that is, if there is more than one affected person. You should see a geneticist.

❖ The presence of an unusual type of disease, such as a male family member suffering from breast cancer, or the presence of several primary tumors in the breast, which is called multifocal.

❖ Having a disease in both breasts at the same time or with a time interval (does not include recurrence of the disease).

❖ Suffering from other primary cancers at the same time or with a time interval (of course, these issues do not include the spread of the disease to other parts of the body or the recurrence of the disease).

If there are one or more of the above cases, the patient should refer to a geneticist to determine the probability of the disease for himself and his family members. Usually, geneticists, after consulting and drawing a family tree, will check for mutations in genes predisposing to breast cancer.

The most common genes that are investigated are breast cancer genes 1 and 2, which are called BRCA2 and BRCA1 for short. All the genetic codes of the affected person are checked for mutations, and if there is a mutation, the disease is not hereditary and we do not need to check others, but if there is a mutation that causes the disease, in the next step, all related people in the family are checked for the presence or absence of genetic mutation is examined.

This means that there is no need for a complete investigation in other members of the family and only the same area where the mutation was observed in the affected person is investigated. Another point is that family members are screened based on inheritance in the family tree. For example, if a person is infected, to check the nieces, the patient's sister is checked first, and if there is no mutation in her, there is no need to check her children.

Hereditary muscular dystrophy diseases

These diseases form a large group of hereditary diseases and are transmitted from parents to children through gene transfer. Some of them have such an obvious manifestation that it appears in all the children of the parents. Duchenne and Becker muscular dystrophy are progressive genetic diseases linked to the X chromosome that cause destruction or disruption of muscle tissue.

Muscular dystrophy includes 8 types of diseases, the prominent and severe example of which is Duchenne and Becker muscular dystrophy, which cripples the patient in childhood. Duchenne and Becker muscular dystrophy is caused by a defect in the X chromosome and lack of dystrophin protein. The gene responsible for making this protein (DMD) is located on the X chromosome.

Limb-girdle muscular dystrophy (in English: LGMD) is genetically heterogeneous, and the clinical symptoms of the disease include the initial weakness of the hip and shoulder muscles, followed by the muscles of the proximal part of the arms and legs. The analysis of the association of genes with the disease in large families and in families with consanguineous marriages showed that mutations in the genes that encode Sarcoglycan proteins are related to this disease. Fascio-scapulo-humeral muscular dystrophy or FSHD is a genetic disease that is transmitted from one generation to another in an autosomal dominant form, and its frequency is 1 in 20,000 people. In this disease, the muscles of the face, shoulder and upper part of the hand are affected first, and then the weakness of the muscles of the pelvis, abdomen and the lower part of the leg occurs, and many patients also suffer from hearing loss. In most cases, the disease begins at the age of 20 or more, and in 20% of cases, the patient moves with a wheelchair at the age of 50. The location of the FSHD disease gene is at 4q35, which is located near the end of the long arm of chromosome 4.

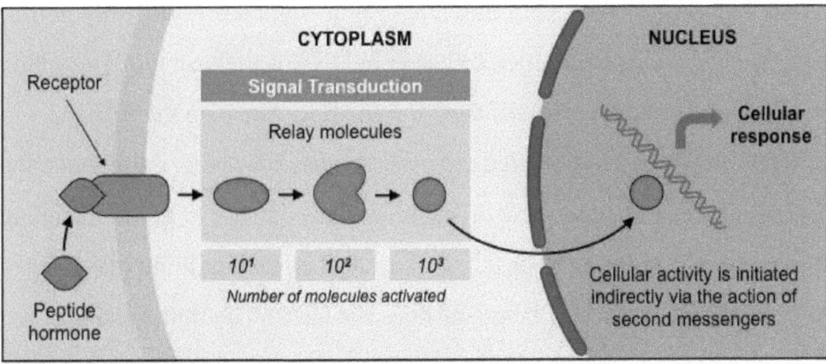

Figure 33. Types of Hormones | BioNinja

Emery Dreyfus muscular dystrophy is one of the types of muscular dystrophy. This disease is caused by a mutation in the emerin gene and a change in the amount and structure of this protein.

The symptoms of this disease include the loss of movement of the muscles of the spine, elbows and ankles. Gradually, other skeletal muscles also weaken, and in the second decade of life, the patient dies of a sudden heart attack. The cause of death is the disruption of the rhythms of the atria and ventricles.

According to the above, we are facing diseases in which the root of life is a problem. Our earthly life is created with a four-letter language of nucleotides in DNA, and billions of different forms have been formed in existence by shifting these nucleotides, increasing and decreasing them, and merging them together. Nucleotide is a compound consisting of a 5-carbon sugar (ribose or deoxyribose), phosphoric acid (phosphate) and one of the bases of allypurine (adenine, guanine) or pyrimidine (cytosine, thymine, uracil). These nucleotides are present in the structure of DNA and RNA.

DNA work in cells

The genetic messages contained in the DNA molecule are ultimately used for such things as making proteins and RNA molecules in the cell. Pieces of DNA that carry genetic messages are called genes, but DNA also has other sequences that are used to make the DNA itself or regulate the use of the genetic information contained in the gene. Cytosine is present in RNA and DNA; While uracil is found only in RNA and thymine in DNA. This four-letter language in DNA is the origin of all proteins and amino acids and thousands of different forms of existence on the planet.

The language with which God created material life has four letters and these four letters are put together and make the words of material existence or genes. Language in the general sense is not Arabic or Persian or English, but anything that conveys the speaker's intention. Perhaps a language does not have an audible meaning, such as speaking with hands and limbs in the language of the deaf or expressing many concepts by a painter on a screen.

It is clear that mixing the letters or words of any language messes up its entire structure. For example, in the Persian language, mixing letters and words does not leave anything comprehensible. Let's assume that the shape of "And" is changed or deleted in Persian language. What will happen? The story of the words of genes and four letters of nucleotides is the same.

A change in one of these letters will mess up all the words or genes and sentences or proteins and sentences or organisms. It is obvious that here we are not facing a microbe or virus that can be killed with a drug, or we are not facing a nutritional deficiency that can be solved by taking vitamins, or we are not facing an immune cell reaction in the body, rather than an anti-inflammatory drug such as corton will fix the problem.

Rather, the root of the words of life and its letters have been messed up, and it is clear that when the root of the existing material existence changes, we cannot expect much improvement by modifying the leaves and branches. Here you have to go to the root and repair it. The story of genetic diseases is a sad story that although many efforts have been made to eradicate them in recent years, they still dominate humans and humans today are unable to treat many of them.

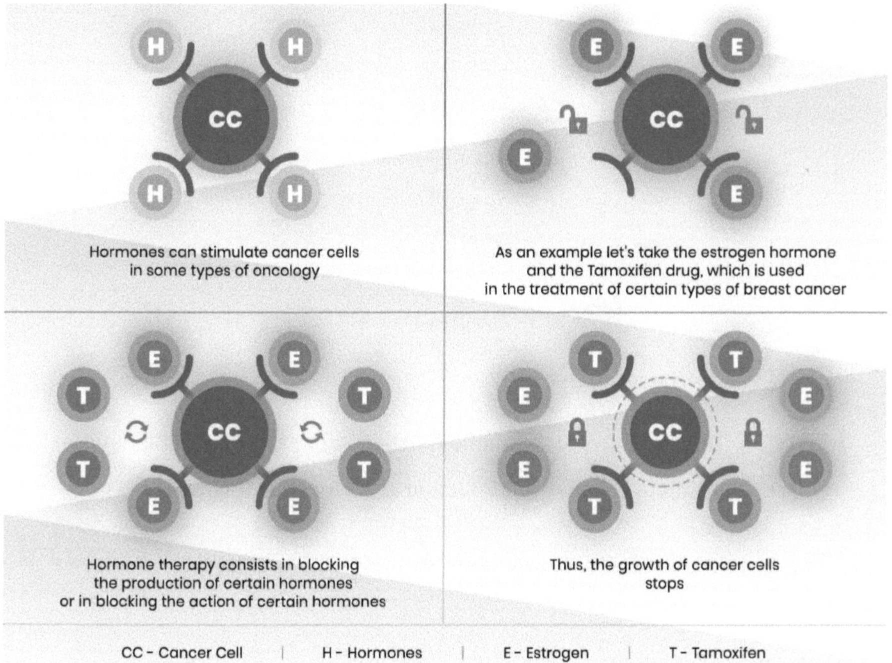

Figure 34. How does hormone therapy work? - High Energy Center

So what should be done?

Being subject to the gene and submitting to it is not limited to these genetic diseases today. There is a bigger genetic disease that humans have inherited from the four ends. A submissive person who today is powerless against the pressure of his sexual genes and gives in to any unhealthy sexual relationship, or the genes in his cells that are similar to those of his genetic relatives force him to always want his children and relatives in the society.

Even if they are guilty, or he is ready to pour various foods into his child's stomach while the stomach of the neighboring children is hungry, or he is indifferent to the voices of children of another race or living in another country, but he is indifferent to the sorrow of the people of his own country or his children. It never goes away and he makes every effort to remove it. This person is suffering from a hereditary disease that he has inherited from all fours.

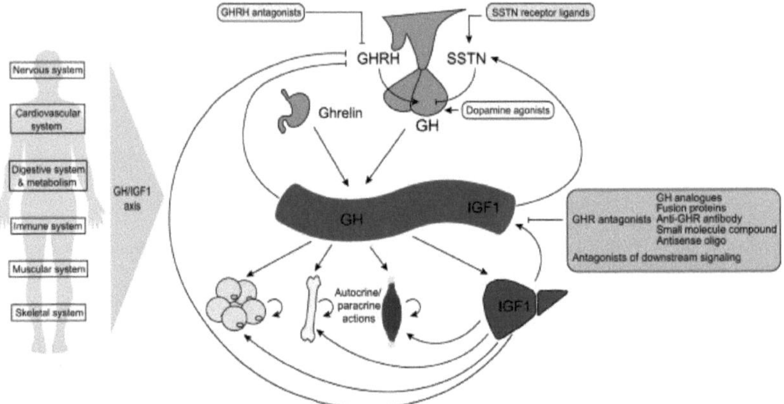

Figure 35. Targeting growth hormone function: strategies and therapeutic applications | Signal Transduction and Targeted Therapy

Chapter V

The role of Hormones in Diabetes and Resilience of People Against it

Diabetes is not only a common disease but also a major health problem that has become widespread in the modern world. Diabetes or sugar disease is a metabolic (fuel) disorder in the body. In this disease, the ability to produce insulin in the body is lost, or the body becomes resistant to insulin, and therefore the produced insulin cannot perform its normal function. The main role of insulin is to lower blood sugar by different mechanisms. There are two main types of diabetes. In type 1 diabetes, the destruction of beta cells in the pancreas leads to the failure of insulin production, and in type 2 diabetes, there is a progressive resistance of the body to insulin, which may eventually lead to the destruction of pancreatic beta cells and the complete failure of insulin production. In type 2 diabetes, it is clear that genetic factors, obesity and inactivity play an important role in a person's disease.

In diabetes, the speed and ability of the body to fully use and metabolize glucose decreases, hence the blood sugar level is increased, which is called hyperglycemia. When this increase in sugar is present in the body in the long term, microvascular complications of diabetes or the destruction of very small vessels are created in the body, which can involve different organs of the body such as kidneys, eyes, and nerves. Diabetic retinopathy is one of the complications of diabetes that affects the eyes. Diabetic retinopathy is seen in three forms: Macular edema (diffuse or localized vascular leakage in the macula), progressive vascular accumulation (micro aneurysm, intraregional hemorrhages, vascular curvature) and retinal arterial occlusion.

Since not controlling diabetes can be associated with serious damage, including damage to the retina, it is very important to investigate psychological well-being and the factors affecting it in diabetic patients with retinal damage. Psychological well-being has been studied abundantly in the research literature in the last two decades, and the scope of its studies has been extended from the field of individual life to social interactions. Psychological well-being, as one of the important aspects of well-being, means striving for transcendence and promotion, which is manifested in the realization of individual talents and abilities, or in other words, striving for perfection in order to realize the real potential abilities of the individual. Various models and opinions regarding psychological well-being have been proposed by psychologists and experts in the field of mental health. One of the most important models for explaining psychological well-being is the model of Ryff and Keys.

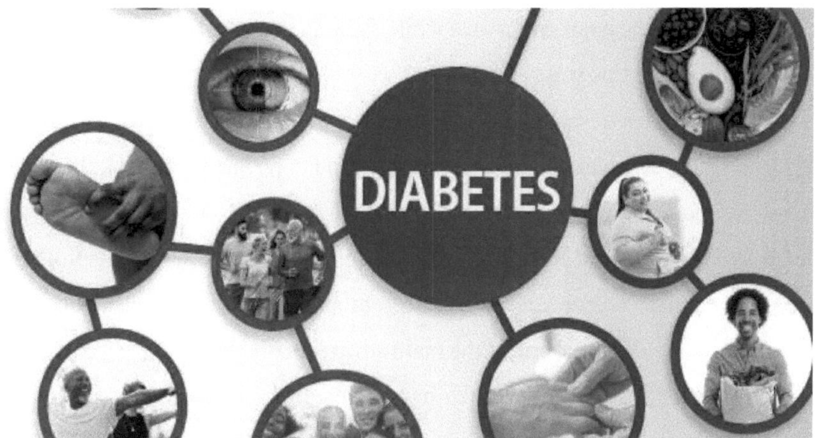

Figure 36. Diabetes Report Card

In this model, psychological well-being is considered as an effort to reach perfection in order to realize one's real potential abilities, which includes six components of self-following, environmental mastery, personal growth, positive relationship with others, purpose and orientation in life, and self-acceptance.

Self-following means acting according to one's own standards and beliefs, even if it is contradictory to the customs and traditions accepted in the society; Environmental mastery means having control over the world around us so that a person can control his life and environment to a large extent; Personal growth includes the ability to flourish all the forces and talents and cultivate new abilities in a person; A positive relationship with others refers to establishing intimate and close relationships with others, while having a desire to establish such relationships, as well as the ability to love those around you; Purpose and direction in life means the ability to find meaning in life and to be purposeful and pursue goals; Self-acceptance also includes a person's positive attitude towards himself, which does not mean narcissism or high self-esteem, but rather self-respect, which is done by knowing one's own strengths and weaknesses. The role of support factors in helping people to actively adapt to stressful events has always been the focus of psychology researchers. So that they believe that in dealing with problems, people can develop more strength and capacity of endurance while fighting stubbornly, so that they can overcome problems in this way.

In the last two decades, researchers have found that people who are successful in dealing with stressful issues and pressures, compared to people who break through problems, have different characteristics and characteristics, in this way, they can withstand less pressure and reach the point as quickly as possible reach spiritual balance. One of these characteristics has been proposed in the form of a concept called resilience. Resilience is one of the main structures of the positive psychology approach. In recent years, this approach has attracted the attention of researchers with the slogan of paying attention to human talents and capabilities (instead of dealing with disorders and anomalies). Resilience includes different concepts.

The term resilience has been defined in various ways: such as the ability to successfully adapt to a changing environment (Darwin, 1989; Cicchitti and Cohen, 1995); Hardiness and invulnerability; and successful adaptation despite high stress and adverse circumstances. But all definitions have a common description and that is "The ability to return to the original state".

Garmezy and Masten (1991) consider resilience as a process, ability or outcome of successful adaptation despite challenging and threatening circumstances. In another definition, resilience means revealing competence in people despite being under pressure and high stress. Rutter (2001) believes that resilience is positive adaptation in response to adverse conditions. Life expectancy as one of the antecedents of psychological well-being has various definitions. Jananche Frankel (1984) believes that when a person engages in his favorite activities, meets others, watches artistic and literary works, or takes refuge in the lap of nature, he feels hope.

Also, when he feels that his existence is connected to a single source, and he considers himself dependent on broad and reliable frameworks and bases such as religion, and he has chosen a philosophy to live, he sees life, understands it and feels it. Considering the importance of examining the antecedents of psychological well-being in diabetic patients with retinal damage, the present study aims to investigate the predictive effect of resilience and life expectancy on the psychological well-being of diabetic patients with retinal damage.

The World Health Organization (2001) defines health as a state of complete physical, mental and social well-being and not merely the absence of disease. In other words, according to this organization, mental health is a state of well-being in which a person is aware of his abilities, adapts to mental pressures, and is productive in his work. Despite the above emphasis on positive issues, health professionals are often so focused on the problems of sick people that they forget the needs of healthy people. According to others, instead of paying attention to the positive aspects of health, mental health centers are more involved in the treatment of mental illnesses (Pilgrim, 1997). Diabetes or sugar disease is a metabolic (fuel) disorder in the body. In this disease, the ability to produce insulin in the body is lost, or the body becomes resistant to insulin, and therefore the produced insulin cannot perform its normal function.

Therefore, diabetes is one of the diseases that threaten a person's health and has a destructive effect on other body organs, including the eyes. One of the eye damages caused by diabetes is known as diabetic retinopathy. This disease directly targets the retina and causes the growth of abnormal blood vessels in that part. Therefore, it causes serious vision problems.

According to what was mentioned, the need to pay attention to the physical and mental health of these patients becomes more obvious. Therefore, knowing the factors that determine people's mental health is one of the most important issues of human sciences in contemporary years. Theories such as Maslow's theories of self-actualization, Rogers' full functioning and adult human or all port's adulthood have accepted and benefited from this basic hypothesis in forming the concept of psychological health. Following the emergence of these theories and the positive psychology movement, which emphasized the existence of positive characteristics and the development of individual abilities in mental health, a group of psychologists have used psychological well-being instead of the term mental health. Because they believe that this word brings to mind most of the positive aspects and in this regard, models such as Jahoda's model, mental well-being model, Diener's model and six-factor model of psychological well-being by Ryff (1989) have been compiled, which define and explain health. Instead of focusing on illness and weakness, psychologists focus on a person's abilities and assets.

Ryff's (1995) model is one of the most important models in the field of psychological well-being. In this view, well-being means striving for independence and advancement, which is manifested in the realization of one's talents and abilities. From this point of view, a person who has psychological well-being has characteristics such as self-esteem, extensive social relationships, a sense of self-efficacy, and a sense of independence. In various researches, researchers have found many factors to be effective on psychological well-being, among which the role of individual, social and family factors can be mentioned. But in particular, some research studies the impactful role of resilience paid attention to psychological well-being.

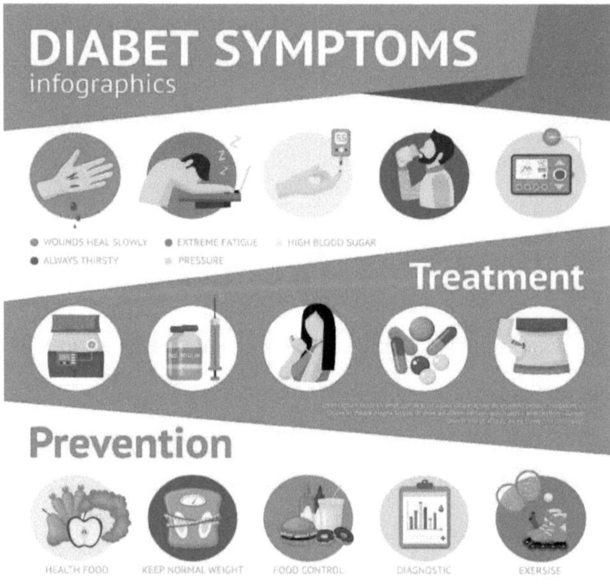

Figure 37. Diabetes patient Vectors & Illustrations

Resilience is a person's ability to establish biological-psychological and spiritual balance against dangerous conditions. Therefore, resilient people are able to maintain their health in different conditions and can experience psychological well-being. Tomas and colleagues (2012) showed in research that resilience is a positive and significant predictor for psychological well-being. Perch, Flanger and Schmidt (2012) found in research that resilience is very important in well-being, so that with increasing resilience, well-being also increases.

Life expectancy is also considered as a mental set based on the mutual sense of will and planning to reach the goal. Therefore, more hopeful people have higher psychological well-being Karreman and Wingerhost (2012) showed in research that people with more hope for the future had the characteristics of re-evaluation, resilience and higher well-being and less repression, but people who were hopeless about the future had lower psychological well-being. Papoulasopoulos and Kepler (2011) showed in research that life expectancy has a positive and meaningful relationship with psychological well-being. However, it should be said that very few studies have investigated the simultaneous predictive role of factors such as endurance and life expectancy on the psychological well-being of diabetic patients with retinal damage. Therefore, the current study seeks to answer the question that are resilience and life expectancy significant predictors for the psychological well-being of diabetic patients with retinal damage?

In fact, the current research aims to investigate the simultaneous relationship of two important individual factors, including resilience and life expectancy, on psychological well-being, in addition to finding the simultaneous relationship of these factors with psychological well-being, the role of each of them in predicting the psychological well-being of diabetic patients. Examine the eye with retinal damage.

The issue of health has been discussed since the beginning of mankind and in many centuries. The World Health Organization considers health to be a state of complete physical, mental and social well-being. Therefore, one of the aspects of health is physical well-being, which is characterized by the absence of physical disease.

Various diseases can have negative effects on public health, so studies have shown that a disease like diabetes can have negative effects on general health and well-being, and in other words, on the quality of life of patients.

Diabetes is one of the most important health problems of developed and developing societies in the present era. Not only the economic losses caused by the existence of the disease in the affected people are of high importance, but the mental and psychological losses caused by it, which are imposed on the sick people and their families, cannot be ignored.

The results of past studies have shown that almost all aspects of the life of patients can be affected by diabetes and cause a decrease in the level of satisfaction and quality of life of patients. The available statistics related to the disease of diabetes indicate that the prevalence of diabetes has increased alarmingly and it has been proposed as a common epidemic of the century.

So that about 135 million people worldwide have diabetes (Fang et al., 2004). In Iran, according to statistics, the prevalence of this disease has varied between 7.3% and 14.5%. Therefore, the importance of investigating diabetes not only as a common disease but also as a major health problem becomes more obvious.

One of the important problems associated with chronic diseases such as diabetes is the occurrence of psychiatric disorders in those suffering from them. Psychiatric factors play a big role in the occurrence of diabetes in susceptible people. Combined attention to psychiatric and medical problems reduces the incidence of complications and increases the quality of life of diabetic patients (Kaplan and Sadock, 1998). On the other hand, one of the topics that has attracted a lot of attention in recent decades is positive psychology.

This point of view emphasizes the capabilities and assets of the individual and believes that the goal of psychology should be to improve the individual's life level and actualize his hidden talents. Today, a new point of view is being formed and expanded in health-related sciences in general and in psychology in particular, which aims to focus on health, well-being, and explaining the nature of psychological well-being.

Psychological well-being has been studied abundantly in the research literature in the last two decades, and the scope of its studies has been extended from the field of individual life to social interactions. Therefore, examining its antecedents is of special importance. On the other hand, in our country, there has been no systematic research on the well-being of diabetic patients with retinal damage.

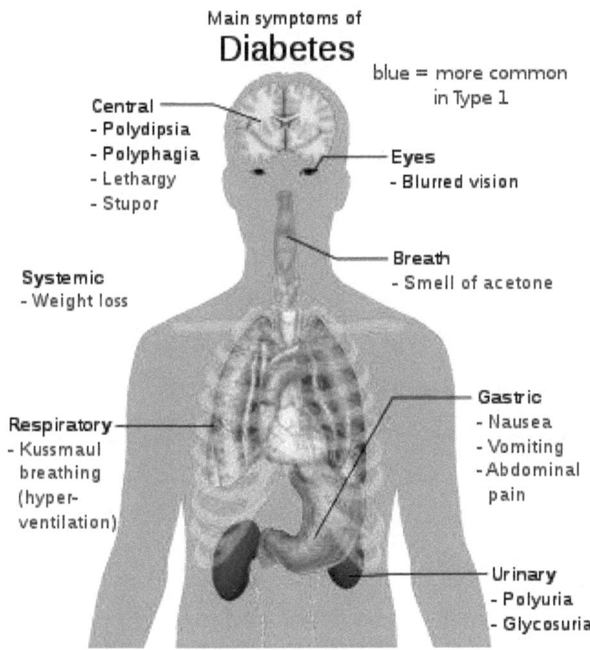

Figure 38. Diabetes

Therefore, it is necessary to pay attention to the level of well-being and its predictive factors in these patients. According to the explanations that were mentioned, it seems that the investigation of the antecedents of psychological well-being in diabetic patients with retinal damage is of considerable importance. A number of researches have investigated family, social and personal factors affecting psychological well-being, among which some researchers have shown that life expectancy and resilience are personal factors affecting psychological well-being.

Definitions of theoretical concepts

Psychological well-being: Psychological well-being is a type of satisfaction and satisfaction of people with the quality of life, which includes a positive state of physical, psychological and social well-being.

Resilience: Resilience is the process of ability or outcome of successful adaptation despite challenging and threatening conditions.

Hope for life: Hope for life is a mental set based on the mutual sense of will and planning to reach the goal.

Diabetes disease: Diabetes is a permanent change in the body's internal chemistry, the result of which is the presence of a lot of glucose in the blood.

Retinopathy (retina problems): Retinopathy is a disorder that causes damage to the retina.

B- Operational definitions

Resilience: Resilience refers to the score that a subject receives from the Conner and Davidson (2003) resilience questionnaire, which includes 25 items and a general dimension, in which the lowest score is 25 and the highest score is 125.

Hope for life: Hope for life is the score that a subject gets from Miller's hope for life questionnaire, which includes 48 questions, in such a way that the score 48 is completely helpless and the score 240 shows the maximum hope.

Diabetic patient: Diabetic patient means a patient who has been treated for diabetes in clinics and medical centers as a diabetic patient for at least one year before.

Diabetic patient with retinal damage: Diabetic patient with retinal damage refers to diabetic patients who suffer from retinal damage and their visual damage has been to such an extent that they need special and accompanying help in their daily life.

Diabetes

The oldest document related to diabetes is the papyrus writings of 1500 BC, in which an Egyptian doctor named Hesira mentioned the symptoms of hyperuricemia and sweet urine for this disease. Hesira treated his patients suffering from hyperuricemia due to diabetes with a special diet including fruits, grains and a little honey. He had no knowledge of the cause of the disease. After him, other Egyptian doctors tried to treat diabetic patients with a similar diet and cucumber flower extract and soaked oats.

About 600 years before Christ, Susrota, the father of medicine in India, described the symptoms of a disease that was later known as diabetes. In the same period, Charaka, one of the doctors of ancient India, called this disease Madhumea, which means honey in the urine. He took help from ants and other insects to diagnose this disease because the urine of people with diabetes attracts ants. Susruta and Charaka were the first doctors to understand that there are 2 types of diabetes. The type that affects thin patients at a young age and the type that affects obese people at an older age. Today's doctors know these two diseases as type 1 diabetes and type 2 diabetes. For many years, many doctors in Egypt, Greece and Rome talked about diabetes and identified this disease until Bu Ali Sina described this disease for the first time in Iran in the twelfth century AD. Since then, scientists have been researching the causes and factors of diabetes and its treatment, and the results showed that some people with diabetes are not able to produce insulin with proper quality.

How does insulin work in the body?

Most of the time, deficiency or complete absence of insulin is the cause of diabetes in young people and adults. The insulin-producing cells in the pancreas of these people are either damaged or completely destroyed. Now it is important to answer this question, how does insulin work in the human body? Consider the human body as a machine; It is clear that our body, like any other machine, needs energy to do work. The three sources of energy in food include sugars and starches (carbohydrates), oils and fats, and proteins (meat, fish, etc.). These substances are finally broken down to produce energy or after decomposition (some of them in the form of glucose sugar) they become storage substances in the liver to be used for energy production in the body later. The most common fuel available to all body cells is a carbohydrate called glucose. Glucose is a simple sugar that is easily consumed by body cells. When the blood sugar rises, the pancreas is stimulated and sends a message through the blood to all the cells of the brain and body. The content of the message is as follows: "The amount of available sugar is high. Use it." This message is the same as the "Insulin" molecule.

Insulin causes a path to open in the cell wall and the received sugar enters it to be consumed or stored. When the blood sugar level is low. The pancreas stops the secretion of insulin. Without insulin, body cells cannot enter sugar. Therefore, they will use fat as a source of energy.

It is during this complex process that the body consumes the food eaten and determines what kind of fuel it has available. In a person with diabetes, the pancreas either cannot secrete enough insulin or the cells are unable to receive the insulin message (like most of the elderly who develop diabetes).

Why should blood sugar be regulated?

In people who do not have diabetes, blood sugar is always maintained at a constant level. Accurate regulation of blood sugar is very important because high blood sugar levels are dangerous. In this case, the kidneys must filter the blood sugar and remove it from the body through urine. In such conditions, a person should drink a lot of fluids to provide enough water to eliminate excess sugar. It is difficult to compensate all the lost water and the body may quickly become dehydrated and this dehydration may threaten the person's life. Cells do not use sugar as an energy source in the absence of insulin. Instead, they are forced to provide the energy needed by the body from another main source, i.e. fat. It is more difficult for the body to consume fat because they are not able to burn it completely. In fact, in the process of breaking down fats, non-consumable substances called ketones are produced in the body. With the increase of these substances in the blood, conditions occur where a person feels dry mouth and stomach pain. If this condition is not diagnosed and not treated with insulin and fluids, it is possible that the person will experience nausea and even lead to death due to heavy breathing and loss of consciousness.

Another danger of being too low is blood sugar. The brain can only use sugar for energy. Therefore, if sufficient sugar is not available, it will send emergency messages to other parts of the body. In this case, the person feels hungry, has a headache, becomes dizzy and loses consciousness, and may even have a seizure. If the blood sugar remains too low for many hours, the brain will suffer serious damage. Therefore, accurate regulation of blood sugar is vitally important and blood sugar should not be allowed to go too high or too low. Although diabetes is called "Diabetes mellitus", it is important to know that when the way of consuming carbohydrates (sugar) in the body changes, the way of using fat and protein inevitably changes. The body's inability to properly use carbohydrates can cause an increase in blood fats, which are sent to the cells as a substitute energy source. Proper diabetes care is actually an effort to improve the natural pattern of food use and energy production.

The concept of diabetes

Diabetes is not only a common disease but also a major health problem that has spread widely in the contemporary world and currently there is no sign of stopping it, but it is increasing sharply. Although a lot of research has been done in recent years on the different epidemiological aspects of this disease, the existing knowledge about its distribution and its determining factors is still insufficient. In recent years, the prevalence of diabetes has increased alarmingly and it has been proposed as the common epidemic of the century. Statistics show that about 135 million people worldwide have diabetes.

In 1996, the World Health Organization conducted a worldwide study to determine the prevalence of diabetes and concluded that in the next twenty-five years, more than twice the world's population will be affected by diabetes, so that it is estimated that by 2025, about 300 will be millions of people with diabetes in the world.

The available documents show a progressive increase in the prevalence of diabetes in most countries, especially developing countries. Pacific and Asian regions are ahead of other countries in terms of diabetes epidemic. About 30 million people with diabetes live in the western regions of the Pacific Ocean. By 2025, fifty million people will be infected in India and China.

In addition, diabetes affects some races more, so that in the last sixteen years, this disease has increased in American Indians and Alaska Natives (Centers for Disease Control, 2003). In the United States, 14.4% (29 million people) of people over the age of twenty have diagnosed diabetes, undiagnosed diabetes, and glucose intolerance (Centers for Disease Control, 2000).

In Indians, the prevalence of diabetes is estimated at 50%, and the lowest prevalence of diabetes is reported in the villages of China and Japan, less than 1% (William and Picu, 1999). In 2000 compared to 1997, the prevalence of diabetes in the United States has increased by 12% (Centers for Disease Control, 2003). Also, the prevalence of diabetes in Bahraini adults is 9% and 17.5% in the black population of the Caribbean.

Several studies report the high prevalence of diabetes in Iran, so that according to studies, the prevalence of this disease has varied between 7.3% and 14.5%.

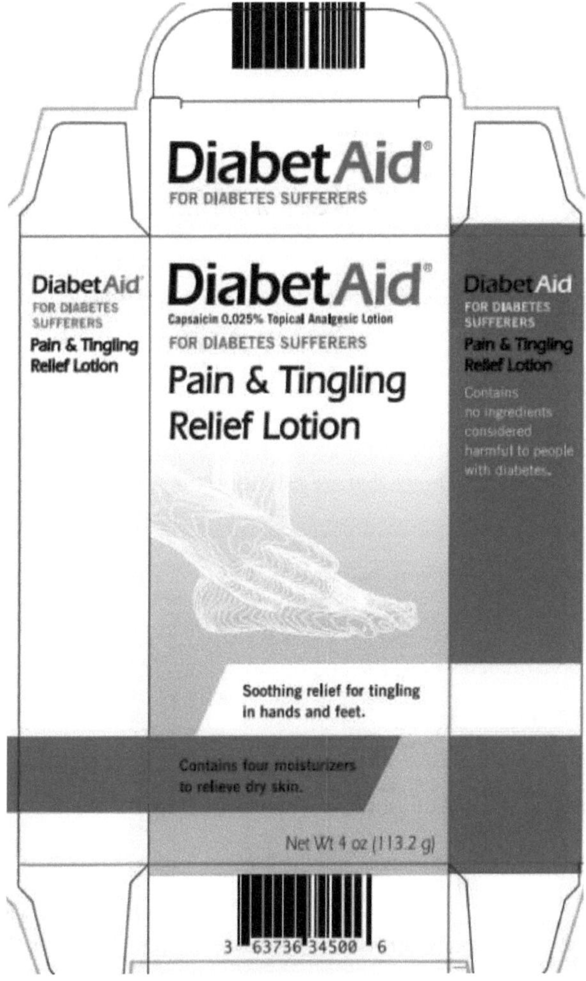

Figure 39. Diabet Aid (lotion) Insight Pharmaceuticals LLC

Also, based on the forecasts of the experts of the World Health Organization, the prevalence of type 2 diabetes in Iran in 1995, 2000 and 2025 will be 5.5, 5.7 and 6.8%, respectively, equal to 1.692.000, 1.977.000. and 5.215.000 people (King, Aubert and Herman, 1998). Diabetes or sugar disease is a metabolic (fuel) disorder in the body. In this disease, the ability to produce insulin in the body is lost, or the body becomes resistant to insulin, and therefore the produced insulin cannot perform its normal function. The main role of insulin is to lower blood sugar by different mechanisms.

In diabetes, the speed and ability of the body to fully use and metabolize glucose decreases, hence the blood sugar level is increased, which is called hyperglycemia. When this increase in sugar is present in the body in the long term, microvascular complications of diabetes or the destruction of very small vessels are created in the body, which can involve different organs of the body such as kidneys, eyes, and nerves.

Types of diabetes

There are different types of diabetes that are usually distinguished during diagnosis. Therefore, determining the type of diabetes depends on the conditions that the disease manifests itself in. In many patients, they do not easily fit into one of the specific categories of diabetes. For example, a person who has gestational diabetes may continue to have diabetes after the end of pregnancy, and therefore the type of diabetes would be changed to type 2.

Therefore, for the doctor and the patient, labeling the type of diabetes is much less important than understanding the cause of this disease and its effective treatment. The old division of diabetes into two types, insulin-dependent and non-insulin-dependent, which was introduced by the National Diabetes Information Group in 1979 and was widely used in the 80s and 90s, caused problems in treatment, which led to the presentation of the classification Diabetes was newly classified by the American Diabetes Association into types:

Type 1 diabetes, type 2 diabetes, other types, and gestational diabetes in 1997. Although this division still has problems, it is used.

Type 1 diabetes: Type 1 diabetes includes two types of diabetes caused by immune reaction and idiopathic diabetes. Immune-mediated diabetes is a heterogeneous disorder caused by known mutations (autosomal recessive and X-linked recessive) as well as polygenic/hypo genic inheritance.

This type includes 5 to 10% of all types of diabetes, previously the term insulin-dependent diabetes or juvenile diabetes was common for this type. In this type of diabetes, cell destruction of beta cells occurs in the pancreas. The main cause of β-cell loss is cell destruction caused by cellular immune reaction. Following this destruction, markers are released in the blood, which include antibodies against insulin, GAD autoantibodies, tyrosine phosphatase 2 IA- and β2IA- autoantibodies. These markers may be seen in 85-90% of sufferers. A connection between certain HLAs and this type of diabetes has also been observed. This type of diabetes is more common in people with DRB gene. The prevalence of this type of diabetes is higher in people who have autoimmune diseases such as Graves' disease, Hashimoto's thyroiditis, and Addison's disease.

In cases of type 1 diabetes, no specific cause has been found for its occurrence, which are classified as idiopathic diabetes. Some of these patients have permanent insulin deficiency and are prone to ketoacidosis, but no evidence of autoimmune reactions is observed in them. A small number of patients with type 1 diabetes are idiopathic, and this condition is more common in African and Asian races. This type is mostly hereditary and not dependent on HLA. The need for external insulin in these patients is not stable and can be transient. In general, in type 1 diabetes, the pancreas does not have the ability to produce insulin, and this substance must be injected into the body at least once a day. This type of diabetes is more common in children and teenagers.

Type 2 diabetes: In type 2 diabetes, which includes 90 to 95% of diabetic patients, the body becomes resistant to the action of insulin. These patients have partial (and not absolute) insulin deficiency at least at the beginning of the disease. This means that the affected person's body produces insulin and the concentration of insulin in the blood may even be higher than its usual amount, but the person's cell receptors become resistant to insulin and in fact do not allow insulin to enter the cells and perform its normal functions. These patients do not need permanent treatment with exogenous insulin to survive. There are several causes for this condition, the partial mechanisms of this condition are not known, but it is clear that autoimmune destruction does not play a role in the occurrence of this disease.

Type 2 diabetes is more common in obese people, and obesity itself creates some degree of insulin resistance. The prevalence of this disease in women is more than men. In this type of diabetes, ketoacidosis rarely occurs spontaneously, but it occurs after a stress such as the occurrence of a disease or infection. This type of diabetes usually remains undiagnosed for years because hyperglycemia (increased blood sugar) develops gradually and is not early enough to show the classic symptoms of diabetes.

However, these patients are exposed to macro vascular and microvascular complications of diabetes. Insulin resistance may decrease with weight loss and drug therapy, but rarely returns to normal. Although the recent increase in the prevalence of this type has been seen in children and adolescents, but in most cases, the risk of this type of occurrence increases with age, obesity, lack of physical activity or an inappropriate diet, and more in women with a previous history of gestational diabetes and people with high blood pressure or blood lipid disorders are seen. Type 2 has a stronger genetic background than type 1, however, the genetics of type 2 diabetes is complex and still not well defined.

Gestational diabetes: Any type of blood glucose increases during pregnancy that reaches the maximum of 5 to 10% of the population is called gestational diabetes. It is known that pregnancy itself can be one of the causes of diabetes. This effect is caused by increasing the body's resistance to insulin and increasing insulin to compensate for this problem. Pregnancy can reveal even mild insulin secretion defects. This leads to glucose intolerance and gestational diabetes. On the other hand, some people who already have a mild blood sugar disorder are classified under this group by screening tests during pregnancy.

Gestational diabetes affects 3-8% of pregnancies and is also one of the risk factors for poor pregnancy outcomes. Also, this condition can independently cause type 2 diabetes. Research has shown that 50% of these women will develop diabetes in the next 20 to 30 years.

In recent years, an increase in the incidence of gestational diabetes has been observed. Several factors have been proposed for this increase. including the high prevalence of obesity in young people, improving the survival of female children whose birth weight is at both ends of the normal birth weight spectrum. In adulthood, these children have impaired insulin function or the ability to secrete insulin, which can make them susceptible to gestational diabetes.

Currently, according to the global statistics and the variables that are effective in contracting this disease, such as the increase in life expectancy, the change in traditional to modern lifestyles, the change in food habits, the amount of physical activity, and the increase in obesity, it seems that it is mature in Iran. More than 3 million people are suffering from this disease, and about 90% of them are type 2 diabetes mellitus (non-insulin-dependent diabetes mellitus), which affects people over the age of 30.

In practice, any person may be affected by diabetes, and this problem does not depend on his age, gender, race or social status. Unlike other diseases such as polio, tuberculosis, and pneumonia, diabetes is not being eradicated, but on the contrary, its prevalence among human beings is increasing every year, and the number of people who get this disease is increasing every year.

Risk factors and diabetes screening

Risk factors and screening in types of diabetes, including type 1 diabetes and type 2 diabetes, are different from each other, which are discussed below.

Risk factors for type 1 diabetes

The risk factors of type 1 diabetes can be estimated by examining the family history of this disease and paying attention to the age of onset and the gender of the family members involved. There are also other ways to predict the occurrence of type 1 diabetes, but since there is still no way to prevent or stop the disease process, the various strategies that exist for the early diagnosis of type 1 diabetes are not of much value.

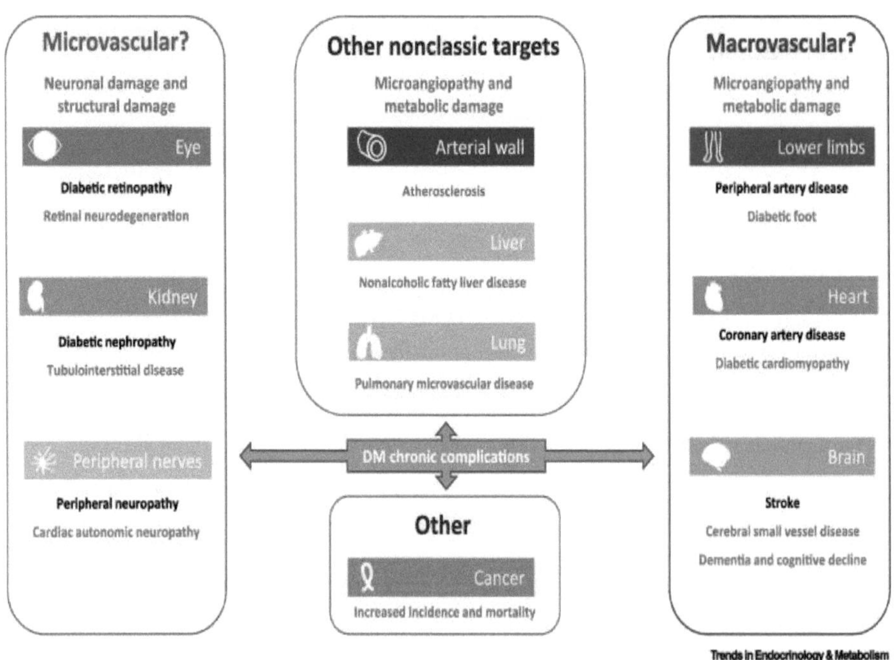

Figure 40. Chronic Diabetes Complications

References

1. Siegel R, Nailshadham D, Ahmedin, J. Cancer statistics, 2012. CA Cancer J Clin; 2012. 62(1): 10- 29.

2. oore MA, Eser S, Igisinov N, Igisinov S, Mohagheghi M, Jarrahi AM, et al. Cancer Epidemiology and Control in North-Western and Central Asia - Past, Present and Future. Asian Pac J Cancer Prev; 2010. 11(Suppl 2): 17-32.

3. Zendehdel K, Sedighi Z, Hassanloo J, Nahvijou A. Improving Quality of Cancer Registration in Iran. Part1: Evaluation and Comparison of Cancer Registration Results in the Country. Hakim Res J; 2010. 12: 42-48. (Persian)

4. Berek JS. Berek and Novak's gynecology. 14th ed. Philadelphia: Lippincott Williams & Wilkins, 2007.

5. Stewart SL, King JB, Thompson TD, Friedman C, Wingo PA. Cancer mortality surveillance-united states, 1990-2000. MMWR Surveill Summ; 2004. 53(3): 1-108.

6. Baig S, Ali TS. Evaluation of efficacy of self-breast examination for breast cancer prevention: a cost effective screening tool. Asian Pac J Cancer Prev; 2006. 7(1):154 -6.

7. Jalalvandi M, Khodadoostan M. Married womwn and PAP SMEAR, what they know? How they do? Iran J Nurs; 2005. 18 (41&42): 139-144

8. Van Laarhoven HW, Schilderman J, Verhagen CA, Vissers KC, Prins J. Perspectives on death and afterlife in relation to quality of life, depression, and hopelessness in cancer patients without evidence of disease and advanced cancer patients. J Pain Symptom Manage; 2011. 41(6): 1048-59.

9. Carter J, Huang H, Chase DM, Walker JL, Cella D, Wenzel L. Sexual function of patients with endometrial cancer enrolled in the Gynecologic Oncology Group LAP2 Study. Int J Gynecol Cancer; 2012. 22(9): 1624-33.

10. Akkuzu G, Ayhan A. Sexual Functions of Turkish Women with Gynecologic Cancer during the Chemotherapy Process. Asian Pac J Cancer Prev; 2013. 14(6): 3561-64.

11. Aarstad HJ, Heimdal JH, Aarsta AK, Olofsson J. Personality traits in head and neck squamous cell carcinoma patients in relation to the disease state, disease extent and prognosis. Acta Otolaryngal; 2002. 122(8): 892-99.

12. Ogden J. Health Psychology. Translated by Kachuie M. Tehran: Arjmand. 2016. (Persian)

13. Nakaya N, Hansen PE, Schapiro IR, Eplov LF, Saito-Nakaya K, Uchitomi Y. Et al. Personality traits and cancer survival: A Danish cohort study. Br J Cancer; 2006. 95(11): 146-152.

14. McKenna MC, Zevon MA, Corn B, Rounds J. Psychosocial factors and the development of breast cancer: A meta-analysis. Health Psychol; 1999. 18(5): 520-31.

15. Persky VW, Kempthorne-Rawson J, Shekelle RB. Personality and risk of cancer: 20 year follow up of the Western Electric Study. Psychosom Med; 1987. 49(5): 435-449.

16. Nakaya N, Tsubono Y, Hosokawa T, Nishino Y, Ohkubo T, Hozawa A. et al. Personality and the risk of cancer. J Natl Cancer Inst; 2003. 95(11): 799-805.

17. Whiteside TJ, Hererman RB. The role of natural killer cells in immune surveillance of cancer. Curr Opin Immunol; 1995. 7(5): 704-710

18. Garssen B, Goodkin k. On the role of immunological factors as mediators between psychological factors and cancer progression. Psychiatry Res; 1999. 85(1): 51-61.

19. Spiegal D, Moore R. Imagery and hypnosis in the treatment of cancer patients. Oncology (Williston Park); 1997. 11(8): 1179-89.

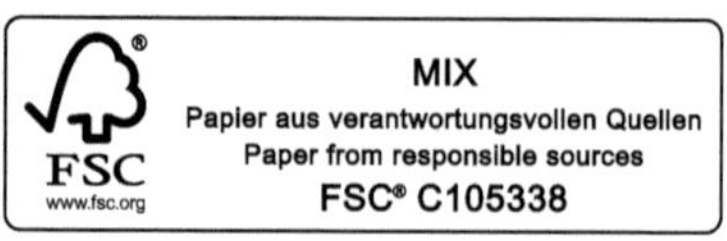

Printed by Books on Demand GmbH, Norderstedt / Germany